Praise for

The 10-Minute Energy [Solution]

"Jon Gordon is a master at teaching people the power of positive energy. If you want to increase your joy and effectiveness as well as your energy level, read this book."   —Ken Blanchard,

coauthor of *The One Minute Manager*® and *Gung Ho!*

"Jon Gordon is a genius when it comes to teaching people how to quickly activate and increase their energy. By reading *The 10-Minute Energy Solution* you will have instant access to a new level of physical, emotional, and spiritual well-being."   —Debbie Ford,

author of *The Best Year of Your Life*

"Drawing upon the latest scientific research, Gordon convincingly makes the case for an evidence-based approach for energetic living. Just reading the book increased my energy!"

—Robert Emmons, Ph.D.,

Professor of Psychology, University of California, Davis

"Jon Gordon knows that true, lasting energy can't be found in a cup of coffee . . . it's all about making smart, simple choices every day. In just ten minutes a day, Jon Gordon can help you transform your life."

—John Gray, Ph.D., author of *Men Are from Mars, Women Are from Venus*

"A fabulous guide for increasing your energy levels and, more importantly, living a healthy, fulfilling life."   —Howard Martin,

coauthor of *The HeartMath Solution*

"Jon's words will inspire you, his authenticity will touch you, and even more importantly, his strategies work! This book will energize your body, mind, and spirit."   —Jeff Keller, author of *Attitude Is Everything*

"Jon Gordon is a mastermind at maximizing positive energy. *The 10-Minute Energy Solution* is a terrific, simple blueprint for incorporating physical, mental, and spiritual lifestyle changes that help you get every ounce out of life!"   —Fran Charles, host of USA Network's *PGA Tour Sunday*

continued . . .

Praise for

Energy Addict

"Simple, powerful strategies . . . Read it so you can go for it."
—Ken Blanchard,
coauthor of *The One Minute Manager*® and *Gung Ho!*

"Your levels of energy largely determine the quality of your life; this book shows you how to feel terrific every minute of the day."
—Brian Tracy,
author of *Change Your Thinking/Change Your Life*

"Jon Gordon's positive energy is contagious. Read this book, get addicted to positive energy, and share it with everyone you know. Someone could say this: Jon Gordon's strategies for boundless energy are right on target for those who want to live a full vibrant life on all levels of their being. Gordon is one of those unique individuals who lives what he teaches."
—Susan Taylor, Ph.D.,
author of *The Vital Energy Program*

"If you often feel like you're out of gas, slowing down, or running on fumes, this book will help you to find the fuel to enliven your life for life. Full of great tips, it's an easy, enjoyable, light, and inspiring read. Jon Gordon's mind-body approach to increasing your energy really works."
—Michael Gerrish, author of the *Mind-Body Makeover Project*
and *When Working Out Isn't Working Out*

"This is the book that people need to read right now. With so many of us needing more energy for our personal and professional lives, this clearly written, practical, and insightful book will make a powerful difference in people's lives."   —Barbara Kaufman, author of *Attitude*

"*Energy Addict* can help many athletes focus and increase their energy during times of high performance. It's been a great book for all my clients who enjoy the game of golf."
—Cindy Reid,
author of *Cindy Reid's Ultimate Guide to Golf for Women*,
and Director of Instruction, TPC at Sawgrass, Top 50 Femal Instructors 2003

The 10-Minute Energy Solution

*A Proven Plan to
Increase Your Energy,
Reduce Your Stress,
and Transform Your Life*

Jon Gordon

America's #1 Energy Coach

A PERIGEE BOOK

A PERIGEE BOOK
Published by the Penguin Group
Penguin Group (USA) Inc.
375 Hudson Street, New York, New York 10014, USA
Penguin Group (Canada), 90 Eglinton Avenue East, Suite 700, Toronto, Ontario M4P 2Y3, Canada
(a division of Pearson Penguin Canada Inc.)
Penguin Books Ltd., 80 Strand, London WC2R 0RL, England
Penguin Group Ireland, 25 St. Stephen's Green, Dublin 2, Ireland (a division of Penguin Books Ltd.)
Penguin Group (Australia), 250 Camberwell Road, Camberwell, Victoria 3124, Australia
(a division of Pearson Australia Group Pty. Ltd.)
Penguin Books India Pvt. Ltd., 11 Community Centre, Panchsheel Park, New Delhi—110 017, India
Penguin Group (NZ), Cnr. Airborne and Rosedale Roads, Albany, Auckland 1310, New Zealand
(a division of Pearson New Zealand Ltd.)
Penguin Books (South Africa) (Pty.) Ltd., 24 Sturdee Avenue, Rosebank, Johannesburg 2196, South Africa

Penguin Books Ltd., Registered Offices: 80 Strand, London WC2R 0RL, England

While the author has made every effort to provide accurate telephone numbers and Internet addresses at the time of publication, neither the publisher nor the author assumes any responsibility for errors, or for changes that occur after publication. Further, the publisher does not have any control over and does not assume any responsibility for author or third-party websites or their content.

PRINTING HISTORY
G. P. Putnam's Sons hardcover edition / January 2006
Perigee trade paperback edition / December 2006

Perigee trade paperback ISBN: 0-399-53290-0

The Library of Congress has cataloged the G. P. Putnam's Sons hardcover edition as follows:

Gordon, Jon, date.
The 10-minute energy solution: a proven plan to increase your energy, reduce your stress, and transform your life / by Jon Gordon.
p.   cm.
ISBN 0-399-15311-X
1. Health.   2. Vitality.   I. Title: The 10-minute energy solution.   II. Title.
RA776.G6555   2006   2005051542
613—dc22

PRINTED IN THE UNITED STATES OF AMERICA

10 9 8 7 6 5 4 3 2 1

PUBLISHER'S NOTE: The recipes contained in this book are to be followed exactly as written. The publisher is not responsible for your specific health or allergy needs that may require medical supervision. The publisher is not responsible for any adverse reactions to the recipes contained in this book.

Most Perigee Books are available at special quantity discounts for bulk purchases for sales promotions, premiums, fund-raising, or educational use. Special books, or book excerpts, can also be created to fit specific needs. For details, write: Special Markets, The Berkley Publishing Group, 375 Hudson Street, New York, New York 10014.

This book is dedicated to my wife, Kathryn.
You are my muse, my inspiration, my love,
my everything. Without you, I would
not be the man I am today. I thank
God for you every day.

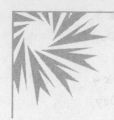

Contents

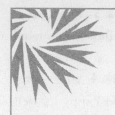

Foreword

Americans are facing an energy crisis of epidemic proportions. More than six million Americans suffer from the devastation of chronic fatigue syndrome and fibromyalgia, and another twenty-five million have disabling persistent fatigue. Beyond this tip of the iceberg, the majority of Americans simply do not have the energy to live the lives that they want to enjoy.

Unfortunately, because these problems only keep you from living satisfactorily (instead of directly killing you), standard medicine pays little attention to them. But my research has shown that both fatigue and pain usually go away or improve markedly with metabolic energy treatments—I call this the SHIN protocol.

Sleep
Hormonal issues (despite normal blood tests)
Infections
Nutritional deficiencies

It is imperative that those with disabling fatigue lay the foundation for physical health by treating these four key areas that are critical for "metabolic health." The SHIN protocol is the physical foundation for creating energy in the cells of your body.

In this wonderful book, Jon builds on these four key areas and gives you practical advice that can boost your energy *now*. Instead of touting the energy boosters in common use—such as caffeine and sugar, which are "energy loan sharks"—Jon gives you advice on how to build sustained and healthy energy. In addition to dealing with metabolism, he recognizes that if he teaches you how to have energy so that you can go back to a life that you hate, he's done nothing for you. He knows that living a life that you hate is a surefire way to quickly drain your energy. He wisely recognizes that having energy serves you best when it helps you to be joyful and happy as well. In doing so, he remarkably ties together physical, mental, and psychological/spiritual truths that are age-old, and yet he's able to present them in a straightforward and easy-to-apply manner.

Joseph Campbell, one of the world's most respected anthropologists, explored spiritual traditions that have existed planet-wide and throughout the millennia. After a lifetime of research, he was asked to summarize his findings. What he answered is an incredibly simple yet powerful truth. It was, "Follow your bliss!" He realized that we have feelings for a reason. Our feelings reflect who we really are. By doing and keeping your attention on things that feel good, you no longer allow the "energy vampires" that Jon speaks about to drain your energy. In the process, you gain the incredible prizes of authenticity and joy, and the abundant energy that comes with these.

Although the three magic words—"Follow your bliss"—summarize what you need to do psychospiritually to gain outstanding energy, it is important that you have a road map that can show you how to get from where you are to where you want to be. The *10-Minute Energy Solution* is such a road map!

It's time for you to get a life you love. As the old saying goes, "If not now, when?" By simply following Jon's advice, you can easily get a life you love *now*. I commend him on his outstanding work!

Best wishes on a powerful and joyful life filled with energy.

—Jacob Teitelbaum, M.D.
Best-selling author of *From Fatigued to Fantastic!*
and medical director of the Annapolis Center for
Effective CFS/Fibromyalgia Therapies in
Annapolis, Maryland, www.Vitality101.com

Do You Have 10 Minutes?

How many times have you been asked this question? Whether it's a friend, a boss, or a coworker speaking, people are always asking us for 10 minutes of our time. And if you are like most people, you always say, "Sure, what can I do for you?" We always make time for others when they need us. Someone wants to bounce an idea off us, we're there. Someone wants to tell us a funny story, we're there. Someone wants help with a problem, we're there. Ten minutes here, 10 minutes there—we are always giving 10 minutes of our time. In fact, we'd probably even give 10 minutes of our time to people who are rude to us!

In the course of our fast-paced, chaotic lives, we give away 10 minutes of our time like free candy to anyone who asks us for a piece—and unfortunately people are not the only recipient of our 10 minutes. Consider all the energy wasters that gobble up our time. Junk mail—10 minutes. Lost keys—10 minutes. Junk e-mails—10 minutes. Waiting in line—10 minutes. Being put on hold—10 minutes. Life is full of 10-minute wasters.

Give Yourself 10 Minutes

Well, now I am asking you to give *yourself* 10 minutes. Instead of spending 10 minutes with someone who drains you, I'm asking you to spend 10 minutes to recharge yourself. Instead of letting life's 10-minute zappers waste your energy, I'm asking you to fill your life with 10-minute boosters that energize you. Ten minutes a day to increase your energy. Ten minutes a day to reduce your stress and increase your happiness. Ten minutes a day to increase your abundance and improve the quality of your life. You may be thinking, "What can I do in 10 minutes?" In this book, I'll show you the power of spending 10 minutes with yourself. Because as you will see, it's not the 10 minutes that matter, but what we do *during* the 10 minutes that means everything.

The 10-Minute Solution

The other day I got a call from my wife. She wasn't happy. "When you get home, you need to weed the lawn. It's overflowing with weeds and you've just been letting it go too long," she said. "So when you get home, you need to get out there and get busy, Mr. Energy." All at once I felt like a little kid again whose dad was making him weed the lawn. I never liked yard work—it just always seemed so hard and overwhelming. And overwhelmed is exactly what I felt when I arrived home and looked at my yard. Denial wouldn't work anymore. Weeds were everywhere and my procrastination was only making it worse. There was no Little League baseball game to run off to. No place I could hide.

As I looked at the yard, I thought, "How am I ever going to get this all done? It's too much. It's too hard." I felt anxious, like someone who is one hundred pounds overweight but doesn't know where to start. I felt overwhelmed, like people who want to make changes in life but don't have a plan. And I felt sad, like a person dealing with depression who sees life as an insurmountable mountain and says, "What's the point?" But then it hit me. I had an insight. *I help people all the time take small positive action steps that produce big results in their lives,* I thought. *Why can't I do that here?* I didn't have to weed my entire yard all at once. I could weed 10 minutes a day, and it wouldn't be hard at all. I went in to tell my wife about the great idea I had. (Let's just say she wasn't so supportive of it at first. I think the phrase "lazy bum" might have been uttered!)

But I put my plan into action. I weeded 10 minutes that day, and 10 minutes the day after, and 10 minutes every day after that until the entire lawn was weeded. It took me only seven days, and it wasn't hard at all. In fact, it was almost effortless. I was amazed at how fast time went by and how much I accomplished by just weeding 10 minutes a day. I felt great. No longer would yard work have power over me. I even started to enjoy the time—I used it to breathe, focus, and relax. Getting control over my life energized me; it gave me a sense of control because I made it a simple, easy, and constant practice.

I realized that we can create and accomplish anything we want in our life by breaking it down into smaller, more doable parts. Just think what your yard would look like if you spent 10 minutes a day for the rest of your life weeding, planting, and gardening. Now picture what your life would look like if you invested 10 minutes a day in your health and happiness over the rest of your life. This is the power of the 10-minute solution. It takes only 10 minutes—but 10 minutes every day over time produces amazing and incredible results.

10 Minutes a Day for More Energy

So maybe you don't have a yard full of weeds like I did. But I'll bet there's something in your life that you'd like to improve . . . if only you had the time and tools to do it. The complaint I hear again and again from people all across the world is that they "just don't have the energy" to make it through their lives. They're exhausted from a demanding job. They're wiped out from dealing with their kids. They don't have the energy to enjoy the things they love most in their lives. I'm here to tell you that life doesn't have to be like this.

Most of us want to have more energy to take on the increasing demands of every day life. Yet, for many of us today, life is more challenging than a marathon—more exhausting than a sprint. It's a constant race that takes its toll on us mentally, physically, and emotionally. Not only are we running to keep up with our to-do lists, but we are constantly hitting detours and roadblocks along the way.

As I talk to people around the country I hear it all the time. They feel beaten up, worn down, and exhausted. In today's time-constrained, energy-strapped society, it is more important than ever to build our energy supply and increase our mental and emotional strength. That's why I wrote this book. With a strong energy foundation we can build mental and emotional muscle that enables us to overcome the challenges of everyday stress, fear, and negativity. We can practice exercises that reduce stress and enhance our happiness and abundance. We can implement a plan that will change the way we think and feel.

But don't just take my word from it. Read on and you'll be able to experience this for yourself. You'll find what the thousands of people who have completed this plan have found. Improving your life and gaining more energy doesn't have to be hard. You can make it simple and powerful. All you need is a foundation and a plan you can fit into your daily life. That's what you'll find inside this book. If you give me just 10 minutes a day for thirty days, I can guarantee that you'll have more energy, less stress, and more happiness in your life.

Chapter 1

What Is an Energy Addict?

Why We're All So Tired—and What We Can Do About It

"I'm exhausted."

As I travel the country, I hear this same lament all the time. People are overstressed, overtired, sleep deprived, and overworked. Does this sound familiar? When I ask in my seminars, "Who here is tired today?" fully three-fourths of the people in the room raise their hands.

Millions are searching for their energy. That's why there's a Starbucks on every corner. It's why energy drinks have become a billion-dollar-a-year industry and why energy bars now take up entire grocery aisles in supermarkets. Yet we know the quick fixes don't work. There are more Starbucks than ever doing more sales than ever, and yet we are more tired and unhappy than ever.

We are like energy vending machines. Every day we are required to dispense energy to our work, our families, and our friends. And let's face it—your kids have a lot of quarters. Your boss or employees have a ton of quarters, and your significant other has a pocketful of change. So the questions you must ask yourself are, "Am I stocked up or sold out? Do I have the energy to give or am I spent?"

Energy Addicts know that if they don't have the energy, they can't share it. They know if they are sold out of energy, they are no good to themselves or the people that matter most. An Energy Addict is aware that energy is the currency of personal and professional success today, so they focus on acquiring more energy for their lives and careers. They know if they stock up their energy vending machine, they will have more energy for themselves and more to share with others. While many people think that energy is just physical, an Energy Addict knows that energy is mental, physical, emotional, and spiritual and it is found in the thoughts we think, the words we say, the music we listen to, and the people we surround ourselves with. In fact, I'll often receive phone calls or e-mails from people asking advice about energy. While we talk I'll often hear something like, "Gee Jon, I thought you were just going to tell me to start exercising and eating breakfast. I didn't know we were going to talk about mental, emotional, and spiritual energy, but I am sure glad we did." I often explain to these people and to the readers of my newsletters and books that energy is more than just exercising and eating right. Energy is everything. You can be in tremendous physical shape but be in the middle of a bad relationship or face a big problem at work and feel emotionally exhausted, which causes you to feel physically exhausted. On the other hand, you can exercise in the morning and this energizes your thinking and helps you take on challenges at work. Or you can focus your thoughts on being thankful and feel your body gaining strength with each dose of gratitude. And if you are like me, when you pray you feel a release of heavy emotional energy from your body. Energy flows in all directions. What we do physically affects us mentally, emotionally, and spiritually, and our mental and emotional state affects our physical state. We are energy beings more than human beings. Einstein's $E=MC^2$ tells us that anything that is matter is composed of energy, and since we are matter, we are energy.

So if we want to improve and transform our lives, we must transform our energy—all of our energy. We must enhance the fuel that we cultivate within ourselves and acquire from the world around us. We must get addicted to positive energy in all its sources; foods that sustain us, thoughts that energize us, emotions that move us, and prayers that fuel us.

Scientists tell us that if we could harness the power within every cell of our body, we would generate enough energy to light up every city in the world. Inside every one of your cells, in every ounce of your energy, and in every bit of your emptiness and nothingness is the energy and power to create anything you want. *You are that powerful*. Energy Addicts know they have this power and they tap this energy from the inside, and they acquire the best sources of energy from the outside.

How I Became an Energy Addict

I feel so passionately about the importance of energy in our lives because having an energetic outlook has actually saved my life. Several years ago, my wife and I got into an argument. It was the most recent of many such disagreements, but this time it quickly escalated . . . culminating in an ultimatum from my wife. She turned to me and said, "Who are you? I don't even know who you are anymore. You are miserable, negative, controlling all the time and you are ruining my life." Then with a look so serious it sent chills down my spine, she said, "If you don't straighten up, I am leaving you. I will not live my life like this. I love you, but I can't live with you like this. I will not spend my life with someone who makes me feel this way."

Talk about a wake-up call. I knew she was dead serious, and I knew I needed to change. My negative energy, unceasing work habits, and constant stress were ruining my marriage and threatening to destroy my family. How did I get like this? I wasn't always this

way. Was it being a young father with two children, a wife, a mortgage, car payments, responsibilities, and pressure out the wazoo that
made me become a miserable, stressed-out, negative man? I would
say they were factors, but in truth, the problem was inside me. When
you press a peanut, you get peanut oil. You don't get olive oil. You
can get only what is inside the peanut. In much the same way when
you are pressed in life, you express only what is inside you. And what
was inside me wasn't good.

When I looked in the mirror, I honestly didn't even recognize myself. Who was I? Where was the happy person who took chances, had
no fear, and lived life to the fullest? Where was the young man who
opened a restaurant at the age of twenty-four and turned it into a
famous Atlanta destination? Where was the guy who started a nonprofit organization to raise money and assist youth-focused chari-
ties? As I looked in the mirror, I knew that this person was still
somewhere inside me. I just had to find him again.

So I asked myself, "What would happen if I was addicted to a
lifestyle that energized me rather than a life that drained me? What
would happen if I was addicted to energy foods that boosted my
moods instead of foods that caused a food coma? How would my life
change if I was addicted to physical and mental exercises that made
me feel great? How would I feel if I intoxicated myself with happiness, fun, positive energy, and trust instead of fear, stress, negativity,
and drama?"

The answers came through loud and clear. I would be happier. I
would be more passionate and purposeful. I would feel less stressed
and be more optimistic. I would create more abundance. I would feel
more powerful, confident, and alive. I would flow rather than struggle through life. I would get addicted to life.

When my wife said, "Change, or I'm leaving," it really woke me
up. Like being shaken out of a nightmare, I woke up, looked at my
life, and knew I needed to make changes. I started reading books
about positive psychology and researched the latest studies in neuro-

science. I spent hundreds of hours researching the connection between nutrition, exercise, mood, and happiness. Then I started making changes in my life. I walked every day. I began lifting weights to build physical muscle and energy. I changed my diet and started eating foods that made me feel great. I worked on my control issues. Several events in my life taught me to let go of control and to surrender to a power far greater than myself. I discovered that trust is the antidote to fear. I learned to forgive those who hurt me, and I started practicing gratitude on a daily basis. I developed exercises to create more happiness, optimism, focus, and positive energy in my life.

And while I was working on myself, I began working with others. I started writing, speaking, and coaching others about what I'd learned in my journey. My speaking and coaching business thrived, and I coined the phrase "Energy Addict" to describe this new lifestyle—I'd become "addicted" to positive energy, and with an almost evangelical zeal I wanted to share my physical and mental transformation with the world.

I wrote a book, *Energy Addict*, in 2003 that shared the 101 physical, mental, and spiritual ways I'd learned to energize my life. The response was tremendous—I appeared on the *Today* show and heard from literally thousands of people all over the world who tried these techniques and reported amazing differences in their lives. I was shocked to learn just how many people suffer from the same symptoms I once did—they're overtired, overstressed, overworked, and overwhelmed. We are all running on empty.

The 10-Minute Energy Solution

My first book, *Energy Addict,* offered an array of 101 tips and action steps you could apply to energize your life. But as I listened to the feedback from my online community of Energy Addicts and spoke with people across the country at my seminars, I realized that many people would also benefit from a more structured plan. People wanted to know exactly what to do and when to do it . . . a blueprint for how to give themselves an "energy makeover" in just a few weeks. So I decided to create a specific Energy Addict plan and share it with my online community to see how it worked. The key was, this plan had to be simple to follow and easy to fit into our busy, stress-filled lives—hence, the "10 Minutes a Day" concept. After hearing about all the positive results and transformations people were experiencing using this thirty-day plan, I decided to write this book with the hope of being able to energize as many people as possible.

It's amazing how dramatic the effects of adding just 10 minutes a day of energizing behavior can be. When I talk about being "addicted" to habits and a lifestyle that energizes us, I'm not referring to a routine of working out at the gym for four hours a day or drinking so much carrot juice your skin turns orange. Rather, I'm picturing you waking up in the morning and looking forward to taking a walk. Not a long walk. Just a short walk that makes you feel great. You take your walk, and as usual it makes you feel rejuvenated, recharged, and refreshed. And this incredible feeling makes you want to do it each day again and again to the point where you get addicted to it in a positive way. Then the benefits of this simple walk cause an energy ripple that improves many other areas of your life. Your life continues to get better and better, and you reach a state where you can't imagine your life, without this positive habit. This walk has become a part of your life, and you have become who you are because of this walk. You have become an Energy Addict and your life will never be the same. I know because it happened to me.

What Drains Your Energy?

So now that you know my story, let's start talking about you and your story. Let's talk about life today and why I believe people like you and me need a plan such as this. Let's talk about why so many people today are so unhappy, tired, and burned out. Then let's talk about ways to reduce your stress and increase your happiness, energy, and abundance. It all starts with identifying the problem, creating a solution, and then applying it to your life. So let's start with the problems.

The Seattle Effect

The first reason why so many people are so tired today is actually a combination of four factors that contribute to one major problem. These four factors include too much technology, too much caffeine, too little sleep, and too little exercise. And when they occur simultaneously in a person's life, you get a modern-day phenomenon I call the "Seattle Effect," named after the place that birthed the new dynamic duo—Starbucks and Microsoft. A perfect combination if ever there was one.

When we used to think of great combinations, we thought of Abbott and Costello, peanut butter and chocolate, Laverne and Shirley. Now, an ideal combination is a double latte and a laptop with a wireless connection. Every generation needs its energy source to grow and build its economy. In the twentieth century it was oil that fueled the industrial age and the trains and steel plants that built our great cities. Today that fuel source is coffee and it's fueling the people who create the digital economy. And there's no other place where coffee and computers go together better than Seattle. Starbucks and Microsoft represent better than any two companies the fuel and the steel of today's world . . . and interestingly enough they are both from Seattle.

And let's not forget the company that made your computer and the Internet one big shopping mall. The company that popularized the Internet and gave you a good reason to spend time at your computer. The name that is synonymous with e-commerce and the Internet—Amazon. And guess where Amazon is from . . . Seattle.

While all this technology and coffee from Seattle is creating our future economy, the problem is that too much of them combined with too little sleep and exercise is draining our energy and destroying the quality of our lives. To my friends in Seattle, please know I don't blame you or your great city. I am simply pointing out that the Seattle Effect, Microsoft, and Starbucks symbolize the problem that is causing America's tired epidemic—a condition I call the T.I.R.E.D. Syndrome.

The T.I.R.E.D. Syndrome

The T.I.R.E.D. Syndrome is a condition in which you feel worse and worse the more you use your computer, your cell phone, and the multitude of electronic gadgets that are supposed to make your life easier. Symptoms include feelings of increased stress, fatigue, depression, anxiety, isolation, and sleep deprivation. The T.I.R.E.D Syndrome stands for *Technology and Information Related Energy Depletion*. I came up with this name after I researched all the medical journals and couldn't find a name that matched technology with these symptoms. It may be a new syndrome, but from all the e-mails I receive and the groups I talk to around the country, I have a feeling that millions of people, like me, have suffered or are suffering from it. If we knew what to call it, we would all be walking around telling each other, "I'm feeling down and I'm pretty sure I have a bad case of T.I.R.E.D." But since it hasn't had a name, we just keep on feeling as if we are in a funk, drinking our double lattes to take on the day—while our condition only gets worse.

It seems every facet of our life is being replaced by electronic substitutes. Instead of exercising we're searching, responding to e-mails, playing online games, and watching television. About 60 percent of adults don't get enough physical activity, and 25 percent don't get any at all. Our physical activity is declining—and the average American spent about 1,669 hours (or about 70 days) watching television in 2004, according to *USA Today*. And instead of getting together with family and friends, we are spending more time on our cell phones and online. Studies show that the average American spends 619 minutes a month on the cell phone and 3 hours a day online. Sure it's great to connect with others online, but you can't hug someone and look into a friend's eyes over the Internet!

Our lives are always on and connected. Whether it's by a phone line, cable modem, cell phone, or PDA, we are always connected to technology and information. We're always plugged in, and instead of drawing power we are expending it, giving it away, or having it sucked from us—costing us our health and our energy. In fact, in a survey of 1,500 people, the HeartMath Institute, a nonprofit research organization, found that the more time the participants spent on a computer, the more likely they were to be depressed.

Are we surprised? Whether it's the dozens of daily e-mails we receive or the countless cell phone calls we take at the grocery store, restaurant, and mall or the continuous incoming messages hitting our blackberry while we are on dates or during playtime with the kids, we are constantly being bombarded with information and distractions—affecting our focus, stress, happiness, and energy levels. Technology is simply moving at a faster pace than our nervous systems can handle.

The T.I.R.E.D. Syndrome begins with a condition I call *buttstickitis totheseatis*: People are simply spending too much time sitting down and not enough time moving. Let's face it, human beings were not meant to sit at computer screens eight to 10 hours a day. We weren't meant to have a cell phone constantly in our ear. We were meant to chop wood and carry water. We were meant to be active, to farm and hunt. Only recently have we become an information-oriented society, centered around computers and technology.

While our way of life has changed our DNA has not, and we just haven't evolved yet to meet these new demands. Information is being transmitted at lightning speeds, and our bodies just want to slow down. But we're not listening, we're not exercising, and we're not finding time for ourselves. After all, there are e-mails to respond to, voice mails to return, and new Google searches to sift through. Instead of technology working for us, we are working for our technology.

It's gotten so bad that I often joke with people in my seminars by giving them a top five list of ways they know they have the T.I.R.E.D. Syndrome. You know you might have T.I.R.E.D. if you are an e-mail addict and get anxious and start twitching if you are away from your e-mail for a day. Or if you chat more online with people around the world than with your neighbors. Or if you named your dogs Google and Yahoo and your child Ebay. Or if you spend more time searching online than you do exercising. Or if you spend more time talking on your cell phone and PDA than with your significant other . . . especially when you are eating dinner! Or if you get bored from sitting quietly in an airport for only a few minutes and reach into your pocket to make a meaningless phone call. Does any of this sound familiar?

A Caffeine Nation

Over time the T.I.R.E.D. Syndrome gets worse, and the Seattle Effect can start to take over our lives. We start to drown in information, being overwhelmed by data and stress, and they are slowly killing us. According to the CDC, more than half of all deaths between the ages of one and sixty-five result from stressful lifestyles. Not a healthy statistic when one in three American employees are chronically overworked and 54 percent of American employees have felt overwhelmed at some time in the past month by how much work they had to complete (Families and Work Institute). It's no wonder that 90 percent of doctor visits are stress related.

At this point in the process of trying to keep up with all the demands of technology and life, we reach a critical point of the Seattle Effect. In order to make it through each day, we fuel up with coffee in order to work more and sleep less. The Seattle Effect has caused us to become a Caffeine Nation—a nation addicted to caffeine to fuel our tired busy lives, a nation that sleeps less and drinks more caffeine in the form of coffee, sodas, and energy drinks. In fact, one-third of Americans get only six hours or less of sleep per night, while sales of energy drinks have soared to over a billion dollars per year and Starbucks made over five billion dollars in sales alone during 2004. Americans are starving for energy, and judging from skyrocketing sales and long lines, they are looking for it in convenience stores and coffee shops selling energy in a cup, bar, pill, and can. Could energy shots at your grocery store be next?

Energy drinks used to be sold in small funky-looking cans. Well, that wasn't enough. Sensing the thirst for energy, now any one of us can receive an energy infusion from huge cans of energy drinks appropriately named "Monster Energy Drink" and "Rock Star Energy Drink." They're loaded with so much caffeine you'll go from slumped to pumped in no time and have the energy to party with the best of them. But if you've seen Ozzie Osborne lately, the important question you must ask yourself is, "Do you really want to party like a rock star?"

The problem with too much coffee and energy drinks is that they are like the energy mafia. They give you some energy when you need it most . . . but you will pay a steep price tomorrow. And that steep price comes in the form of your health and energy. At a time when so many of us are stressed and overwhelmed, the overconsumption of caffeine is just one more reason why we are stressed out and burned out. In a study of seventy-two habitual coffee drinkers, researchers at Duke University found that subjects produced more adrenaline and noradrenaline and had higher blood pressure on days when they drank caffeine compared with days they abstained. "The two stress hormones are vital to helping the body react quickly in times of danger or stress, but they can damage the heart over a lifetime of heightened production," said James Lane, associate research professor of psychiatry at Duke.

It's no wonder the Chinese symbol for busyness is a combination of two other symbols—"killing" and "heart." Lane also said, "Moderate caffeine consumption makes a person react like he or she is having a very stressful day. If you combine the effects of real stress with the artificial boost in stress hormones that comes from caffeine, then you have compounded the effects considerably." Chronic stress caused by anxiety and caffeine also leads to fatigue, headaches, and poor sleep. It's a dangerous combination because lack of sleep is associated with increased drowsiness, inability to function during the day, and decreased quality of life.

In fact, two of the main predictors of whether someone is likely to be depressed is (1) They are not getting enough sleep, and (2) they are not getting enough exercise. What happens next? Since you sleep less, you feel more tired. So you turn to caffeine to wake you up throughout the day, which provides the quick fix you need but also increases the production of your stress hormones. This affects your sleep so you sleep less and feel more tired and around and around you go on the caffeine energy roller coaster—and so begins the vicious cycle that is fueling our technology-driven fast-paced way of life but also causing us to be so tired.

When you add in the fact that people are not exercising, in addition to drinking too much caffeine and not sleeping, you get the entire picture of the Seattle Effect. An ironic twist here is that if more people would exercise, this would reduce their stress, increase their energy, enhance their health, and help them sleep better. But what I hear from so many people is that they are so tired they don't have the energy to exercise and create more energy. One woman told me the other day that she didn't even have the energy to come to my energy seminar. And in many cases people feel like they are so busy trying to keep up that they don't have time to exercise. So they don't exercise and they don't receive all the benefits that exercise produces.

The fact is, sustained energy cannot be bought in a bottle and we cannot replace sleep with a double latte. While a can of espresso may help you take on the day, it will certainly impact you tomorrow. We cannot keep our engines running on overdrive and not expect to burn out. Just as the world must look for other fuel sources besides oil, we must find real and sustained sources of energy to fuel our tired lives. And we must manage our fuel consumption by not scattering so much of our energy with so much technology usage.

I'm not saying we shouldn't use technology. We simply must become smarter about how we use technology. And I'm not saying that people shouldn't drink moderate amounts of coffee for enjoyment or start their day with a cup of coffee. If you love your morning cup of coffee, I say have it and enjoy it. My rule of thumb is, "A morning cup of coffee, good. A morning pot of coffee, bad." Coffee isn't evil. But relying on caffeine for our energy is hazardous, and we should stop consuming so much of it.

Instead of caffeine addicts and technology addicts, we need to become Energy Addicts. Instead of scattering our energy, we must learn to focus it. Instead of acquiring sources of energy that drain us, we must get addicted to positive, powerful, and sustained sources of energy. Instead of our body relying on caffeine for energy, we must tap our natural power sources that are available to us every day. And best of all, these power sources are cheaper than a four-dollar cup of coffee, much more healthy than a can of "Monster Energy," and provide more sustained energy than a can of Diet Coke. The rest of this book will offer the solution to counter the Seattle Effect and heal the T.I.R.E.D Syndrome. Consider it a T.I.R.E.D cure filled with strategies you need to fuel up with the best, most powerful, and sustained sources of energy.

The Stress Factor

Not only is stress a byproduct of the Seattle Effect, but it is also a stand-alone cause of why we are so tired and burned out. As I mentioned earlier, more than 90 percent of doctor visits are stress related, and stress is linked to six of the leading causes of death: heart disease, cancer, lung illness, suicide, cirrhosis of the liver, and accidents. Iron-ically, stress was meant to be our friend, helping us run faster and fight harder to ensure survival. It all has to do with the fight-or-flight response, which is hardwired into our ancient DNA. If you have ever faced a scary or stressful situation, you know what it's like to feel the fight-or-flight response. Our blood pressure increases, we produce more stress hormones, and more blood sugar and oxygen are pumped through our body to keep us alert and ready.

The fight-or-flight response was essential to our survival in a bru-tal and primitive world. It helped us run faster to get away from ani-mals chasing us. It helped us fight harder when we needed to survive. However, now we don't often face many life-threatening situations that require us to "fight or fly" anymore. Let's face it, these days most of our stressful and fearful situations come from life and career pressures—a new project deadline, an argument with a coworker, running late while taking the kids to soccer practice. Instead of chopping wood and carrying water as our bodies were meant to do, we now sit at desks for twelve hours a day. Instead of battling oppos-ing clans for power and control, we're battling the competition for business. Instead of searching for food to eat, we are searching for happiness. Our fight-or-flight response system that helped us survive during the stone age now slowly kills us during the information age.

Whereas in the distant past we might have experienced fight-or-flight responses occasionally and used up the stress hormones by fighting or running, many of us now live and work in office environ-ments in a constant state of fight-or-flight—with elevated amounts of stress hormones coursing through our bodies. And as we once al-lowed our bodies time to recharge and refuel after a stressful event, now we are in a constant state of red alert in a chronic state of stress—which is wreaking havoc on our mental and physical health. Chronic stress weakens our immune system, increases our blood pressure, accelerates aging, affects our energy levels and sleep pat-terns, and depletes the neurotransmitters dopamine and serotonin that make us feel happy—creating a vicious cycle of fatigue, burn-out, anxiety, and depression.

Short-term stress is our friend and helps us run faster, work a lit-tle harder, and accomplish a little more. Chronic stress is clearly pub-lic enemy number one. Instead of fueling up with calm energy, we are fueling up with too much stress energy.

The Sea of Negativity

We live in a sea of negativity. Whether it's the newspaper, twenty-four-hour news stations, or radio, we are constantly being bombarded by negative news, negative images, and negative energy—and it's taxing our mental, physical, emotional, and spiritual energy. Negativity has become so common we don't even realize it anymore, yet if we really pay attention and read between the lines and listen behind the words, it's as if someone is shouting, "Fear, fear, fear," into our ears.

The root cause of all stress is fear. Like stress, fear is ingrained in us and throughout our history it helped us survive. Fear of starving caused us to search for food. Fear of being attacked caused us to pro-tect ourselves. Even today fear helps us. Fear of getting hit by a car causes us to look both ways before crossing a street. Fear of being at-tacked in a strange neighborhood causes us to be alert and look over our shoulder. Fear asks the question, "What can I do to stay alive?" Fear wants to know, "What can I do to protect myself?" These ques-tions cause us to be more alert and on guard.

The media knows this, and they know that people respond to fear—so this is what they serve us so we will tune in and listen. So they can have higher ratings. So they can sell advertisements to com-panies that sell antidepressants that we need . . . because of all the sadness we feel from reading, hearing, and watching all the negativ-ity! It certainly is a vicious cycle that leads to a constant state of fear for many. Not only do we have to worry about keeping our job and putting food on our table, but now we must be reminded every day that terrorists want to blow us up. We must be told of all the horror in the world, and yet we never hear about the millions of random acts of kindness that happen every day around the globe. Unfortunately good news doesn't sell. And the news that does sell penetrates our senses. It fills our ears with negative stories and our eyes with horrific images. It seeps into our soul, filling it with pain and despair.

Just spend half an hour watching one of the twenty-four-hour news stations. Then write down how you feel. How does your body feel? Anxious? Tense? Do you feel uplifted or pessimistic? Living in a sea of negativity is like being surrounded by ice-cold water. It causes you to get tense, freeze up, and resist the natural flow of life. We are clearly being bombarded with too much negativity and fear, and over time it slowly drains us of our joy, happiness, and positive energy.

The Energy Vampires

As I wrote in my book *Energy Addict,* energy vampires lurk in our families, organizations, neighborhoods, and companies. They are everywhere, and we are all exposed to them like germs. When you are in the presence of an energy vampire, you know it. If you pay attention, you can almost feel them sucking your positive energy and life force from you. You feel like a balloon that's just been deflated. They don't do it with fangs but rather with negative energy that acts like a big positive energy vacuum.

Energy vampires are fearful so they share fearful energy. They are often miserable so they share their misery. They are negative so they share negative energy. I don't condemn energy vampires; nor do I want to hurt them with a stake or garlic. (They'll smell you coming a mile away . . . and tell you how badly you stink!)

With so much negative energy in the world, it's no wonder that so many people have been infected with energy vampiritis. I think of my own past and understand that there are times that I have been an energy vampire. We all have. Just remember that the people you surround yourself with have a huge influence on your energy. And more important, your ability to deal with the energy vampires that surround you in your life is one of the most significant factors that contribute to your overall happiness, health, and emotional well-being. Later in the book we'll discuss specific ways to stop the energy vampires from sucking your energy.

Plastic Food

Another main source of our energy drain is plastic foods. Think about it. Your body recycles the food you eat to create the building blocks that make up your muscles, brain cells, blood cells, and heart. Your body knows what to do with things that come from nature. It knows how to process and recycle a banana, water, fish, or carrots. However, it has no idea what to do with diet soda, hydrogenated oil, food colorings, and man-made processed foods that have ten or more ingredients with words you can't pronounce. Just as an engine can't run properly without the right fuel, you won't operate as efficiently or effectively without the right energy foods.

Unfortunately, many of us are relying on very inferior sources of energy when our busy lives demand we operate at peak performance. Instead of eating eggs and fruit for breakfast, we're eating doughnuts. Instead of water, we're drinking soda with aspartame. Instead of eating foods that grow on farms, we're eating too many things manufactured in plants. Our body doesn't need dead food. It needs live food—whole food that comes from nature. It doesn't want Fruit Roll-Ups. It wants fruit.

Consider that in every health magazine there's always a new research study demonstrating the benefits of whole foods such as blueberries, walnuts, avocados, garlic, and tomatoes. We may read that one food has a certain property that fights cancer, while another food contains an active ingredient that boosts our mood. Again and again we hear about the positive link between whole foods, health, happiness, and energy, and yet we never read that toaster pastries help build strong bones or fluorescent orange cheese puffs are great for your heart. Our approximately one hundred trillion energy cells need real, live energy to grow and thrive, and it's no wonder that we are tired from a processed, fake-food diet. Fueling up with plastic and processed foods devoid of real nutrients, essential fats, and vitamins that our bodies need to stay energized is taking its toll on our mental, physical, and emotional health. Later in the book, we'll discuss what foods you should be eating to boost your energy, increase your happiness, and enhance your health.

Emotional Pain

We all have it. It's part of life and part of the human drama. For some reason we must go through pain to find a deeper meaning and higher understanding. But while we are going though our pain, it's difficult to see the bigger perspective. And if we have allowed emotional pain to accumulate over our lifetime, then it's even harder to see above the clutter and feel our way out of our accumulated emotional fat. When too much emotional pain accumulates, life becomes emotionally exhausting and draining. Even minor setbacks cause you to experience a cascade of negative emotions, fear, and stress. Emotional pain weighs you down and makes you feel as if you have a hundred pounds of rocks in your pocket. Unfortunately, if left unchecked, these rocks can grow and get heavier. In addition, new pains arise and add new rocks to your pocket, all taking its toll on your mental, physical, emotional, and spiritual health. Thankfully there is a way to let go of the rocks that weigh you down. That's what this plan is all about.

Hidden Energy Drainers

Hidden energy drainers include a variety of conditions that a majority of people are not informed about. When I coach people, I first have them go through an audit to rule out these hidden energy drainers as a cause of their fatigue, unhappiness, or burnout. Several of these hidden energy drainers include:

➤ Chronic fatigue syndrome and fibromyalgia

➤ Hepatitis C

➤ Food allergies

➤ Anemia

➤ Multiple chemical sensitivities

➤ Hypothyroidism or hyperthyroidism

➤ Sleep apnea

➤ Multiple sclerosis

➤ Diabetes

While a book could be written about each one of these conditions and many books are, I present this list to you so you are informed and can see your doctor, have blood work done if necessary, and make sure these conditions are not the cause of your lack of energy. If you do have one of these conditions, you can conduct research and take specific steps in association with this plan to improve your health. Helpful research resources include: www.endfatigue.com, www.drweil.com, www.webmd.com, and www.prevention.com.

10-Minute Energy Solution Energy Audit

The purpose of this assessment is to help you identify which energizing habits you possess and which aspects you need to improve. To maximize your benefit from this evaluation, I suggest you not only evaluate yourself but also have your family, friends, coworkers, or colleagues evaluate you. Have them do it anonymously to make it more honest and powerful.

Step 1—Rate yourself or have someone rate you on each quality, characteristic, and habit below.

Step 2—Tally the score. Use the Energy Meter to gauge your energy level.

Step 3—Identify your areas of strengths and weaknesses.

Step 4—Use the action steps presented in this book to improve your weaknesses.

Step 5—Evaluate yourself every three months to track your progress and improvements.

From 1 to 10, how would you rate your . . .

	SOMETIMES		**OFTEN**
Physical energy	Appears physically vibrant and energized		
	1 2 3 4 5 6 7 8 9 10		
Water intake	Drinks enough water to stay hydrated and energized		
	1 2 3 4 5 6 7 8 9 10		

		SOMETIMES								**OFTEN**	

Diet   Eats whole foods from nature, not processed foods

1 2 (3) 4 5 6 7 8 (9) 10

Exercise   Makes time for daily exercise

(1) 2 3 (4) 5 6 7 8 9 10

Silent energy   Takes time for silence to reduce stress

1 2 3 4 (5) 6 7 (8) 9 10

Positive energy   Feels positive and shares positive energy

1 2 (3) 4 5 6 7 (8) 9 10

Optimism   Possesses and displays an optimistic attitude

1 2 (3) 4 5 6 7 8 (9) 10

Happiness   Enjoys life and work: smiles often

1 2 (3) 4 5 6 7 (8) 9 10

Gratitude   Gives thanks often and freely

1 2 3 (4) 5 (6) 7 8 9 10

Play   Has fun at work and in life

(1) 2 3 4 5 6 7 8 (9) 10

Confidence   Believes in oneself

(1) 2 3 4 5 6 7 8 9 (10)

Trust   Learns and grows from challenges and mistakes

1 2 3 4 5 6 7 (8) 9 10

Mental muscle   Ability to overcome negative people and situations

1 2 3 4 5 6 (7) 8 9 10

Empathy   Ability to genuinely empathize with others

1 2 3 4 (5) 6 7 8 9 10

Compassion   Expresses genuine concern for others

1 2 3 4 5 (6) 7 8 9 10

	SOMETIMES	**OFTEN**

Being present   Engaged with work and others in the moment

1   2   3   4   5   6   7   (8)   9   10

Magnetism   Ability to attract the right people

1   2   3   4   (5)   6   7   8   9   10

Contagious energy   Ability to connect with others

1   2   3   4   (5)   6   7   8   9   10

Hospitality   Ability to make others feel welcome and comfortable

1   2   3   4   5   (6)   7   8   9   10

Listening   Listens genuinely and actively

1   2   3   4   5   6   7   (8)   9   10

Openness   Is open and accessible to others

1   2   3   4   5   (6)   7   8   9   10

Enthusiasm   Demonstrates enthusiasm for life and work

1   2   3   4   5   6   7   (8)   9   10

Passion   Expresses passion at work and in life

1   2   3   4   5   6   7   8   (9)   10

Purpose   Knows mission and works toward it daily

1   2   3   4   5   6   7   (8)   9   10

Vision   Sees it, embraces it, and works toward it

1   2   3   4   5   6   7   (8)   9   10

Forgiveness   Ability to let go of anger and resentment

1   2   3   (4)   5   6   7   8   9   10

Balance   Makes time for family and people that matter most

1   2   3   4   5   6   7   (8)   9   10

Self-care   Takes time for oneself to recharge and reenergize

1   2   3   4   (5)   6   7   8   9   10

Self improvement   Takes time to grow, develop, and improve

1   2   3   4   5   6   7   ⑧   9   10

SCORE TOTAL _208_

ENERGY METER
TOTAL SCORE

1	75	150	225	300

TIRED	YOU'RE ON YOUR WAY	FULLY ENERGIZED
This plan is the fuel you need now	Take your energy to the next level	Keep doing what you are doing and use this plan to grow and improve

Chapter 2

Your 7 Essential Energy Boosters

How You Can Create a Foundation of Positive Energy in Your Life

I have a friend who brings inner city children to watch sky-scrapers being built. He does this to help children learn that before they can start building the structure, they must first dig, and dig, and dig to create the foundation. In fact, they dig for months before they do anything else. The children realize a profound fact of life: You can't grow and you can't build if you don't have a foundation. They learn that you must first go down deep before you grow. As adults, we must learn this same lesson. If we want to grow and transform our energy, we must first create a foundation that will support our growth. Once we create a solid and strong foundation we can grow as high as we can dream.

The key words here are *strong* and *solid* foundation. As someone who lived through three hurricanes in Florida in 2004, I noticed that all the fast-growth trees were knocked down by the strong winds, while the larger trees, the ones that took years and years to grow, were still standing. The trees that took the longest to grow had the strongest roots—and the roots held the trees up. I realized in our lives we have to develop a strong root system or foundation of powerful lifelong habits, not quick fixes, that will sustain us when the winds of life blow. These habits don't provide a strong root system over night, but with practice and repetition they will build your energy and your life one day at a time.

Your Energy Foundation

So this plan starts with creating your energy foundation. Instead of living a life filled with energy drainers, my goal is to help you create a foundation of energy boosters—simple positive habits that help you think clearly, act energetically, and live optimally. As I have coached thousands of people, I have found one of the most basic, overlooked problems is that so many of us are not doing the little things that create a solid energy foundation. We have become so busy and stressed that we have forgotten the basics. Thus this foundation is about bringing back the basic principles of energy into your life, and these simple energy boosters will make a world of difference.

The great thing about the habits I am about to share with you is that you are already doing them. They include eating, drinking, sleeping, breathing, listening, and moving. Now, I just want to help you do them optimally, powerfully, and effectively. After all, you may be eating, but you may be eating foods that tear down your foundation instead of building it. You may be drinking, but you may be drinking fuel that clogs up your energy system. And you may be sleeping, but perhaps not enough to sufficiently recharge your batteries.

At first these habits may feel awkward, like wearing your watch on your other wrist, but over time these strategies will become a part of you. When you are down, they will help lift you up. When life and work are chaotic, they will provide a strong foundation to help you withstand the storm. When you are faced with obstacles and challenges, this foundation will keep you standing strong in the face of adversity and help you proceed on your path to success. Life is not easy and work can wreak havoc on your mental, physical, and emotional energy, but with this plan you will be equipped with the tools to sustain your energy, enhance your happiness, and build success one day at a time.

Your life is the result of the hundreds of daily habits you do each day. Research suggests that 95 percent of your habits are automatic. So when you create an energy foundation of daily habits that increase your energy you will create a more energetic life. Aristotle said, "We are what we repeatedly do. Excellence, therefore, is not an act, but a habit." So if you want to enhance your focus, happiness, energy, and success, I encourage you to incorporate these seven energy boosters into your life and let the habits and action steps create your life. The power of this plan can be realized only if you take action and unleash it.

The foundation you are about to learn is the foundation I have used to dramatically improve my life and become a better father, writer, teacher, husband, and person. It is the foundation I have used to help people from all walks of life feel more alive. In fact, I wrote about a number of these habits in my first book, *Energy Addict*. I wanted to feature the key energy boosters again for those who haven't read that first book yet, and also to serve as a reminder for those who have.

While many of these tips are the same suggestions our moms have been giving us for years, I encourage you not to be fooled by their simplicity. We often have a tendency to overlook the simple things. We believe they are too simple to have such a big impact and yet from the thousands of people I have coached and all the success stories I have received, I know that small changes produce big results. Make these habits a part of your energy foundation even just for the next thirty days and witness the benefits for yourself. So let's start creating your energy foundation one bite, one breath, one gulp, one snore, one step at a time.

Your 7 Biggest Energy Boosters

Energy Booster #1: Get More Sleep

While there is a mountain of research and evidence that demonstrates that a lack of sleep negatively impacts our mood, stress levels, alertness, weight, ability to process glucose, performance, and reaction times, we really don't need to know the research in order to understand how we feel when we don't get enough sleep. Sleep is truly tied to every facet of your life, and if you don't get enough sleep, nothing else will work very well. As I wrote earlier in the book, you can't replace sleep with a double latte. A lack of sleep is one of the main reasons why people are so tired today, and sleeping more is one of the best ways to boost our energy. According to David G. Meyers, author of *The Pursuit of Happiness,* happy people live active, vigorous lives, yet they reserve time for renewing sleep and solitude. So get some sleep and get happy.

Since there are many conflicting studies on how much someone should sleep, when people ask me, I say, "Sleep until you feel great." Each person is different, and while some people truly need only four hours a night, most of us need between seven and eight hours. To determine how much sleep you need, consider the following rules.

Sleep Tips:

➤ Do your own energy experiments and determine how much sleep you need to feel your best. Go to bed a little earlier each night to see how much sleep makes you feel the most rested in the morning.

Jon's Energy Rules

➤ If you have to rely on caffeine to wake you up during the day, you are not getting enough sleep

➤ If you wake up tired, you are not going to bed early enough

➤ If you feel sluggish during the day and you eat an energizing diet and you exercise, you are probably not getting enough sleep

➤ Get a TiVo, tape your late-night shows, and get the sleep you need to operate at peak performance.

➤ Make your sleep time a ritual. Every night go to bed at the same time.

➤ Nap for twenty to thirty minutes for a rejuvenating and recharging power nap if you did not get adequate sleep the night before. Research demonstrates the power of a power nap, and it is an amazing way to reenergize during the day if you can find the twenty to thirty minutes and a comfortable place to do it. Research shows that any longer than thirty minutes can make you more tired, so stick to twenty to thirty minutes when napping.

Energy Booster #2: Move Your Body

When you're active you feel like you can move mountains. As you probably already know, exercise is one of the best things you can do to increase your physical and mental health. Research shows it is as effective as Prozac for people with moderate depression. But as you probably also know, many of us are not exercising like we should. I know what you are probably saying: "But, Jon, I don't have the time," or "It's too hard." Well, my answer is that we must make the time, and it doesn't have to be hard. You don't need expensive equipment or a gym membership. Just get your shoes on and go for a walk. Get moving and get walking. Even 10 minutes will make a difference. Just do some form of exercise each day. Here are some more simple ways to make exercise an important part of your energy foundation.

Exercise Tips

➤ Don't hit that snooze button. Get up earlier and increase your metabolism and energy by exercising first thing in the morning.

➤ If you don't have a dog, get one and take her for daily walks.

➤ Read a book while riding an exercise bike. You'll be increasing your mental and physical energy at the same time.

➤ Start dancing again. It's a great way to move and energize. Make one night a week your "go out dancing" night.

➤ Work your way up. When beginning an exercise routine, start with small easy steps. When you start small, you realize how easy it is and how great it makes you feel. Then you get addicted to the exercise in a positive way. Over time 10 minutes turns into fifteen minutes, and fifteen minutes turns into thirty minutes. Before you know it, you are exercising forty-five minutes to an hour a day and it has become a key part of your energy foundation and your life.

➤ If you feel time is your daily enemy when it comes to exercise, break your exercise down into smaller parts. For example, try walking 10 minutes in the morning, 10 minutes after lunch, and 10 minutes after dinner. Research shows that three 10-minute walks produce the same health benefits as one thirty-minute walk.

➤ Vary your exercise routine. Keep it fresh and fun. Walk one day; ride a bike the next. Also try jumping rope, purchase a stationary

bike if you can afford one, or try a home exercise video. I offer
several on my website, www.jongordon.com.

➤ Move with yoga. It's not just for Madonna. Millions of people
are benefiting from yoga and you can, too. Again, if you are too
busy and don't have time to attend a yoga class, don't let this
stop you from receiving the health benefits that come from practicing yoga. Buy a yoga video and do your own simple yoga class
for as much time as your schedule permits. If you have only five
minutes, then simply do five minutes of yoga. Start when you can
and stop when you can. Just doing a little something every day
will produce big results over time. For a great selection of yoga
videos visit www.gaiam.com

Note

Make sure you consult with your doctor before beginning any
yoga or exercise routine.

Energy Booster #3: Breathe for Energy

Whenever you feel stressed, breathe. It's one of the simplest ways to
replace stress energy with calm energy. When we get stressed, we take
shorter more shallow breaths, which affects our oxygen intake and
energy level. Something goes wrong at work? Breathe. You have a
challenge at home? Breathe. You notice that you are not breathing at
your desk? Breathe. Feeling stressed while driving in your car?
Breathe. Simply focus on your breathing. Concentrate on inhaling
for two seconds, then exhaling for two seconds. Take five to 10
breaths or as many as you need to feel calm again. As you are breathing, think of a mantra, such as " I feel great," or "life is good," or
"Thank you, God." Breathing is an instant energizer that can be
done anywhere, anytime. Try this for a week and it will become part
of your energy foundation for the rest of your life.

※

Breathing Tips

➤ When you are working at your computer, pay attention to your breathing. We tend to hold our breath when we work intensely. Make the word "Breathe" your screensaver on your computer.

➤ Whenever you are at a red light in your car, use this time to close your eyes and breathe. As Wayne Dyer says, "Someone will let you know when your time is up."

➤ Breathe in some peppermint. Researcher Dr. Bryan Raudenbush of Wheeling Jesuit University in West Virginia found that inhaling peppermint improves an athlete's mood and motivation. Well, you don't have to be an athlete to take advantage of peppermint. Just get some peppermint oil or a peppermint inhaler—yes, they really do make a peppermint inhaler—and wake yourself up at home or at work with 100 percent natural peppermint. I use it and love it.

Energy Booster #4:
Drink the Ultimate Energy Drink

In a world of energy drinks and caffeinated beverages, water is the ultimate energy drink. Research shows that a lack of water consumption leads to fatigue and headaches, and unfortunately most of us are walking around dehydrated without realizing it. Even a small decrease in your weight causes a significant drop in your energy level. The human body is made up of about 70 percent water; not Diet Coke or double lattes. So water is the fuel source you need for increased energy and enhanced health. Every one of your body's processes is enhanced with proper hydration. Digestion improves, your metabolism increases, and your blood flows easier. Think of water as the oil your engine needs to make everything run properly.

So how much water should we drink? While we all have heard the eight eight-ounce glasses per day rule, this is actually a myth. Each person, based on weight and activity levels, requires different amounts of water. To determine how much water you need, convert your body weight into ounces; then divide by two. Thus, a one hundred pound person would convert their weight into one hundred ounces. Then they would divide by two. So a one hundred pound person would need fifty ounces of water a day to stay hydrated. Those who exercise must drink even more water, depending on how much you perspire during your workouts. For a free water calculator, visit my website, www.jongordon.com. Once you know how much water you should be drinking, you can use the following tips to drink more water.

Hydration Tips

➤ Drink a cup of water when you first wake up in the morning. With each sleeping breath you expel water, so this will replenish the water you lost through the night.

➤ Sip water every ten to twenty minutes throughout the day. This keeps you alert, hydrated, and energized. A little water at a time adds up to a lot over the course of a day.

➤ For even more energy drink ice-cold water. Studies by Dr. Darden, the director of research for Nautilus Sports/Medical Industries in Colorado Springs, demonstrates that a gallon of ice-cold water requires more than 200 calories of heat energy to warm it to core body temperature of 98.6 degrees. Thus, this heat energy that your body creates to warm the cold water provides you with more energy for your life.

➤ Carry a bottle of water with you in your car and take water into business meetings. This will keep you hydrated during drives and long meetings.

➤ Drink water instead of soda, juices, and energy drinks. You'll feel the difference.

➤ When you feel hungry, drink water first. We often mistake thirst for hunger. We eat when what our body really wants is water. When you drink water first, you'll eat less and lose weight.

➤ For my favorite water, visit www.pentawater.com. It tastes so clean and fresh it makes you want to drink more water.

Energy Booster #5:
Eat for Energy

Eating for energy means eating more whole organic foods that come from nature and less processed foods. These foods include fruits, vegetables, nuts, legumes, fish, hormone-free and antibiotic-free chicken, beef, and tofu. When we eat real food that comes from nature, we feed our body the energy it needs to operate at peak performance. For thousands of years we ate whole foods. Our bodies know how to process them. However, only in the last forty years did we start consuming large amounts of chemicals, pesticides, and plastic foods manufactured by man instead of nature. Let's face it. Your body knows how to process an apple, but it has no idea what to do with a Fruit Roll-Up. Each one of your approximately one hundred trillion cells needs energy to survive and thrive. By feeding your cells live, whole foods, you provide them with live energy that enhances their health, vibrancy, and operation. Your metabolism increases, your energy rises, and your mental and physical health improves. Start eating the foods you were born to eat and you will feel the difference.

Jon's Energy Rule

Eat more foods that grow on trees and plants and fewer foods manufactured in plants.

Eat Whole Foods

As you eat more whole foods and fewer processed foods, you'll also want to choose organic whole foods when possible. Not only is it better for the environment, but it is better for you. Certified organic crops are not genetically engineered or modified, irradiated, or fertilized with sewage sludge. They are grown as they were meant to be grown—without pesticides, herbicides, and any other chemicals. Just the other day I had an organic orange and a conventionally grown orange side by side. I ate both and it was amazing how much juicier and tastier the organic orange was.

More important, they are also healthier. Organic food tends to contain higher levels of natural cancer-fighting antioxidants and essential minerals such as calcium, magnesium, iron, and chromium. A University of California, Davis, study of organically grown corn, strawberries, and marionberries found that they contained higher levels of natural cancer-fighting compounds than conventionally grown samples. The study reported that pesticides and herbicides used in conventional farming appear to impede the production of phenolics, which defend plants from insects and people from disease.

Organic eating is also beneficial because standards prohibit the routine use of antibiotics and growth hormones in farm animals, which humans ingest when they eat meat or chicken. When eating

Jon's Energy Rule

Eat food with as few chemicals, pesticides, and toxins as possible. Like a river craves fresh running water, our natural bodies prefer clean, healthy food that makes us feel great.

meat, you should choose brands that are hormone and antibiotic free. Yes, they are a little more expensive, but our health is worth it.

Eat Breakfast

In addition to eating whole foods, another key factor in eating for energy is when you eat, how often you eat, and the size of your meals. For instance, you'll want to start your day with more energy by eating breakfast. When you don't eat breakfast, your body goes into energy conservation mode. It says, "I don't know when I'm going to eat again; I'd better conserve energy." So your body produces less energy and you have less to expend. When you eat breakfast, your body says, "Okay, I have the fuel and now I can get moving." Your body produces more energy and therefore has more to spend. Various studies show that breakfast eaters are more productive and alert at work and have more energy in the morning. Breakfast eaters also tend to maintain their ideal weight and are less likely to binge on high-fat high-calorie foods at night. For breakfast you'll want to eat protein and fiber, both of which slowly release sugar into your bloodstream and supply you with sustained energy. Fruit and eggs or hummus are good examples. Here are two of my favorite energizing breakfasts.

Bowl of Energy

Stonyfield Farm Low-fat Plain Yogurt
Chopped walnuts
½ cup old-fashioned oatmeal
½ cup pineapple or 1 apple
¼ cup blueberries

This is a flexible recipe. Use all or a few of the above ingredients, depending on what you have on hand and what you like.

1. Spoon a few tablespoons of yogurt in a bowl. Spoon as little or as much as you like.
2. Add ½ cup of old-fashioned oats. You will want the yogurt to soak up the oats to make them soft. You can do this at night, cover and put in the refrigerator, or in the morning before you exercise and/or shower.
3. Cut up a pineapple or apple into chunks. Cut big or small, whichever you like.
4. When you are ready to eat, add the pineapple or apple and blueberries to the yogurt.
5. Add the walnuts. They are a great source of protein and omega-3 fatty acids (the good fat).
6. Eat and energize.

Energy Cocktail

1 banana
1 cup blueberries (organic fresh or frozen)
    or Sambazon Acai berries
1 apple
1 tablespoon peanut butter, almond butter,
    or ground flaxseeds, or ¼ cup walnuts
    if you have a Vita-Mixer.
1 scoop Earth's Promise Greens
    from Enzymatic Therapy
1 cup soy milk or milk
1 cup of ice

Blend in a blender or Vita-Mixer

For more energy you'll also want to eat smaller, more frequent meals instead of one to three large meals. Studies show that if you eat moderate-size meals plus small between-meal snacks, you in-

Jon's Energy Rule

Eat breakfast like a king, lunch like a prince, and dinner like a college kid with a maxed-out charge card.

crease your levels of energy and alertness. Without healthy snacks, your blood sugar falls and you experience fatigue and tension. According to William Nagler, M.D., psychiatrist at the University of California, Los Angeles School of Medicine, evidence indicates simple hunger-related tensions contribute to fading energy, negative emotions, and late-day arguments. We are like an energy furnace, and we need to continually supply our internal furnace with food that can be turned into fuel. This keeps our mind and body strong and steady. And contrary to how Americans eat, we need to eat more like the French and eat our biggest meal first and our smallest meal last. Studies from the University of Minnesota show that those who eat a majority of their calories earlier in the day and have bigger breakfasts and smaller dinners have more energy.

High-Energy Foods

While you are eating breakfast and smaller meals throughout the day, you'll want to make sure you eat high-energy foods that boost your mood, your energy, and your brain health. Eat these high-energy foods and remember to stay away from processed foods such as candy bars, refined flour, refined sugar, cookies, and food made in factories.

High-Energy Omega-3 Essential Fatty Acids: They are called essential because your body doesn't make them. You must obtain them from your diet. The problem with omega-3s is that we are not consuming enough of them, and this is affecting our mental health, according to many health experts. The bottom line: We need to consume more omega-3s. Considering that the brain is 60 percent structural fat and the brain synaptic membranes and connections, where much of the communication traffic and neurological function happens, is composed of a large portion of essential fatty acids, it's no wonder that omegas are so important to mood and brain health. With fewer omega-3s, the brain cells cannot communicate properly. Health experts believe a diet rich in omega-3 can help improve the communication between brain cells. In fact, according to Dr. Stoll, increasing omega-3s has a direct effect on serotonin levels, a neurotransmitter known for its "feel good and happy" qualities.

So where do you get your omega-3s? Try these sources.

➤ **Wild Alaskan salmon:** Loaded with DHA and EPA, it's a great source of omega-3 essential fatty acids. Make sure your salmon is wild Alaskan and not farm-raised, which contains high levels of cancer-causing toxins—PCBs. Other fish that contain omega-3s include sardines, herring, and tuna.

➤ **Walnuts:** Walnuts contain the plant-based omega-3 alpha-linolenic acid (ALA). Chop and sprinkle on salads, cereals, and oatmeal, or grab a handful for an energizing snack in the afternoon.

➤ **Flaxseeds:** These contain alpha-linolenic acid as well. Grind with a coffee grinder and keep refrigerated in a tightly sealed container. Grind only a week's worth of flaxseeds at a time so they don't go rancid. Sprinkle a teaspoon on cereal, oatmeal, or add to a smoothie.

➤ **Fish oil:** For those who don't eat enough fish, you may want to try supplementing your diet with fish oil. Fish oil is a major source of omega-3s EPA and DHA. One brand known for quality and purity is Nordic Naturals (nordicnaturals.com).

High-Energy Veggies

Every day it seems a new study comes out reporting the benefits of a different vegetable. Whenever I hear this, I chuckle because it makes perfect common sense that vegetables would provide us with the benefits of health and great energy. While I could write an entire book on the benefits of eating vegetables, the goal is to eat a variety of vegetables throughout the week. From broccoli and spinach to tomatoes and onions, here are a few high-energy vegetables I love.

Amazing Avocados: They are high in fat, but it's the good, mono-unsaturated fat. Your brain and body need great sources of fat and research shows that we need to eat the good fat to burn the bad fat. Plus, avocados are a great source of folate, potassium, and fiber. Fiber is essential to maintain energy throughout the day and also fights cancer and protects your heart. Add a few slices to your sandwich or make guacamole.

Definitely Do Dark Leafy Greens: They are loaded with anticancer compounds, vitamins, and minerals. They are a great source of Vitamin B_9 (folic acid), beta-carotene, and vitamin C and fiber. Examples include collards, spinach, and asparagus. Other vegetables that are excellent for your energy and health include broccoli, considered the most nutritious vegetable and also a great source of calcium, red peppers, green peppers, and onions.

Garlic Is Great: Not only does garlic keep the energy vampires away, but research suggests that it also keeps colds and cancer away. Garlic is antibacterial, antiviral, antifungal, and protects against cancer and heart disease. Studies show that when you put garlic in a petri dish filled with bacteria, all the bacteria die. This makes sense when you understand that garlic used to be given as an antibiotic before antibiotics were created. After reading about all the health benefits of garlic, I started eating it frequently. As someone with two small children who always had a cold, I can say that I have not had a cold since I started eating garlic. I have been so amazed with the benefits of garlic I have been spreading the garlic gospel. Even my wife, who was making fun of me for eating garlic, has noticed that I have stayed healthy while everyone around me was getting sick. She is now a garlic fan and has experienced the benefits as well. Every few nights and at the onset of a possible cold we eat three cloves of garlic. We mince it in a food processor or garlic grinder and add it to either apple sauce (I got this idea from Dr. Andrew Weil) or tomato/veggie juice. We go to bed, exercise in the morning, and by the time I'm around people, my garlic smell is gone.

High-Energy Fruits

As with vegetables, the goal is to eat a variety of fruits during the week. Eat fruits with breakfast and as a midmorning or afternoon snack. Here are a few high-energy fruits that will enhance your energy.

Be Berry Happy with Blueberries: They have ten times more antioxidants than almost all other fruits and vegetables. They are also a "good carbohydrate," meaning that they release sugar into your blood at a slower rate and maintain your energy level.

Bananas: They are chockful of vitamin B_6, which facilitates the body's production of serotonin.

Overjoyed with Oranges: Great source of folic acid, fiber, antioxidants, beta-carotene, and vitamin C.

Run with Raisins: Raisins provide you with potassium—a mineral your body uses to convert sugar in the blood into energy. I like to eat raisins with nuts as an afternoon snack.

Acai Berries: Imported from the Amazon rainforest by the company Sambazon (www.sambazon.com), these Brazilian palm berries, which taste like a blend of berries and chocolate, are considered a near-perfect fruit. They have monounsaturated fat similar to olive oil; protein and amino acids similar to egg whites; even more antioxidants than blueberries; and more flavonoids than red wine. Talk about a high-energy fruit.

High-Energy Protein, Legumes, and Nuts

Foods with protein and fiber help us to sustain our energy and blood sugar level throughout the day. In addition, they give us the healthy nutrients and minerals we need to build a strong body and mind. Here are several high-energy protein sources.

Get Enthusiastic About Eggs: They are what nutritionists call a near-perfect food and complete protein (because of all the essential amino acids eggs contain), which are low in saturated fat and loaded with Vitamins A, D, B$_{12}$, folic acid, riboflavin, phosphorous, iron, and zinc. Look for organic eggs that contain omega-3s in your supermarket.

Peanut Butter or Almond Butter: Great as a snack on whole-grain toast or with an apple.

Get Nuts: A great source of vitamins, minerals, protein, Vitamin E, and monounsaturated fat. They're fattening only if you eat too many of them. Eat a handful a day to increase your energy and health. Walnuts are a great source of omega-3 essential fatty acids. Almonds are considered the super nut, with the best combination of monounsaturated fat, protein, and vitamin E. Brazil nuts are a great source of selenium. The *Journal of the American Medical Association* found that those men who consumed the most vitamin E from food sources and not supplements had a 67 percent lower risk of Alzheimer's disease than those eating the least amount of vitamin E. Try different nuts and see which ones you like. You can buy chopped nuts and add them to cereals and salads. You can eat them as a snack in the afternoon when you need a sustained energy boost, or you can liquefy them using a Vita-Mixer, as I do, and add them to smoothies. This is great for kids.

Say Yes to Yogurt: Yogurt (low fat, with live cultures) provides calcium that helps you absorb other vitamins and nutrients into your cells, boosts your immune system, fights bacteria, and helps keep your intestinal tract healthy. Look for a yogurt that is organic and not filled with sugar and sweeteners. I recommend Stonyfield Farm yogurt.

Fresh Home Made is the best!

Go Gonzo for Garbanzo Beans: Aka chickpeas, they are rich in the best source of fiber—soluble fiber—so they help to eliminate cholesterol from the body. Chickpeas are an excellent source of protein, folate, vitamin E, potassium, iron, manganese, copper, zinc, and calcium. Simply add to a food processor—and a little oil—to make healthy and delicious hummus.

Get Bear Naked: Check out my favorite breakfast cereal and snack mix for a healthy all natural serving of nuts and oats—www.bear naked.com.

High-Energy Chocolate Treat

Now you don't have to feel guilty. Dark chocolate really is a health food . . . in small amounts, of course. It's tasty, delightful, and smooth . . . and by now we have all heard about the antioxidants, phenols, and flavonoids found in dark chocolate that may improve heart health. But did you know that dark chocolate also contains a number of chemically active compounds that can improve your mood and pleasure by boosting serotonin (the happy neurotransmitter) and endorphin levels in the brain? So when you are feeling down, don't grab for the Twinkies. Grab a piece of dark chocolate instead. Of course, this doesn't mean dark chocolate should be a staple in your diet, but when it's time for a treat, you'll feel good about making it dark chocolate. Look for a brand that has at least 56 percent cacao.

High-Energy Vitamins

While it would be great if we could get all of our vitamins and minerals from whole-food sources, we know that this is not always possible. So supplementation is recommended for enhanced health and energy. Talk to your doctor about taking these vitamins.

Multivitamin: Health experts suggest we take a vitamin that contains about 100 percent of the RDA (recommended dietary allowances) for most vitamins and minerals. A multivitamin ensures that you are getting enough vitamins and minerals to maintain your health and energy.

B-Complex: This is traditionally made up of ten B vitamins, such as B_1, B_2, B_3, B_5, B_{12}, folic acid, etc. The B vitamins help support the clearing of stress hormones by the liver, enhance energy metabolism in the body, and help keep the nervous system healthy, among other benefits. New research also suggests that the B vitamin folate is needed to build important substances in the brain—a lack of which may cause depression and other mental disorders. B complex vitamins come in various strengths—B50 (which means 50 mg of each B vitamin), B75 (75 mg of each B vitamin) and B100 (100 mg of each B vitamin).

Coenzyme Q-10: Coenzyme Q-10 (CoQ10) is an essential component of the energy-producing machinery of the body's cells. CoQ10 can be compared to a spark plug in a car engine. Just as the spark

Essential Information About Vitamins

➤ Look for a vitamin that is made with the natural food source instead of synthetically. Look for product terms such as whole-food supplements.

➤ To determine which strength and combination of vitamins are right for you, talk to your doctor or health practitioner. Experienced and knowledgeable people who work in health-food stores are also a useful educational resource.

➤ Remember, vitamin supplements should not be used to replace a healthy diet but should be incorporated into one. The best source of nutrients, vitamins, and minerals comes from healthy whole foods.

plug provides an initial spark to start the engine, CoQ10 also kick-starts energy production within your cells, especially in the heart cells.

Energy Booster #6: People

It's a simple rule of life called the elevator principle. There are those who bring you up and those who bring you down. As we go through life we must be mindful that the people we surround ourselves with have a tremendous impact on our energy level. While learning how to deal with people who drain our energy is an important lesson in life and one that will be enhanced by reading the rest of this book, we must also build our energy foundation with people who support us and energize us. We must make time for people who make us feel great. We must connect with others who give and receive positive energy with us. And we must build a team of supporters that provides us with the fuel we need to take on the challenges of everyday life. Here are a few tips to create an energy foundation of positive people in your life.

1. Make a list of people who increase your energy. Decide who is going to be on your energy-building team. Perhaps it's your boss, coworker, sibling, spouse, parent, or friend. Schedule time with these people each week. You might get together once a week with a friend or mentor for breakfast or lunch. Or you may get together with a group of friends each week. Or you may call your energizers once a week on the phone.

2. Share your goals and vision with your supporters. Ask for their support as you make positive changes in your life. Even better, decide to make positive changes together with your energizers.

3. Start a positive energy club and organize a weekly gathering of positive people where you discuss positive things, read positive books, and engage in positive acts. Many positive energy clubs have been started in various communities by people who have read my books and newsletters and at various companies where I have

spoken. Now it's your turn. E-mail me and let me know when you start a club. You can contact me at jon@jongordon.com

4. Remember to connect with the people who energize you and connect often.

5. Don't forget to make time for your pets as well. While they may not be considered people, they do energize us. Many studies have been conducted that show that pets can enhance our health and happiness. When I was growing up, my dog was my best friend, and I still think about her to this day.

Energy Booster #7: Music

Anyone who has ever had a smile come over their face as they listened to their favorite song on the radio knows the power of music to boost our mood and energy. Music is energy that vibrates with a certain frequency just as every one of our body and brain cells vibrate. When we hear music, we also feel it at a cellular level and this boosts our mental, physical, and emotional energy.

Music is such a powerful force in healing that hospitals are hiring Don Campbell, author of *The Mozart Effect,* to design music for different parts of the hospital that create a certain mood and desired energy effect. For example, in an article in *Spirituality and Health Magazine,* Campbell said, "Music with a tempo that is below heartbeat or with heartbeat is more likely to relax the listener while music with an upbeat (faster than heartbeat) tempo is more likely to stimulate and energize." Music can supercharge us, relax us, and inspire us. The key is to use music in the way you need it and when you need it. Make it a part of your energy foundation and it will serve you for the rest of your life. Here are several tips to help you get energized with music.

Music Tips

➤ When you need an energy boost, listen to your favorite song that adds a kick to your step.

➤ Listen to calming music to help you unwind from a difficult day
at work.

➤ Listen to Mozart to boost your brain development and creativity.

➤ Listen to classical music to create calm energy. Dr. Raymond
Bahr, M.D., director of coronary care at St. Agnes Hospital in
Baltimore, Maryland, said, "Half an hour of music produces the
same affects as 10 milligrams of Valium," according to an article
in *Spirituality and Health Magazine*.

This concludes your seven energy boosters that make up your energy foundation. Now that you have the ingredients to build your
energy foundation, the next step is to grow your energy and build
upon this foundation with the power of the 10-Minute-a-Day Plan.

Chapter 3

The Power of the 10-Minute-a-Day Plan

The Benefits of Following the Plan

As any good coach knows, vision is essential to creating success. If someone has a vision for their life, nothing can stop them from achieving it. One study that showed the importance of "vision" to success was conducted with two groups of engineers and airplane designers. One group was told that they were building the fastest, newest, most innovative airplane ever designed. They were shown a model of the finished product and final design. The other group was just told that they were designing an airplane, and each person was instructed to work on his or her particular area of the design without knowing what they were ultimately building. The study showed that the group who knew what they were building and saw the vision of their design worked twice as long, twice as hard, and finished much quicker than the other group.

So with this in mind, I want you to understand the larger purpose of this 10-Minute-a-Day Plan. I want you to know what this energy plan is designed to help you do. I want you to know the reason behind the 10-minute exercises and the results they will help you achieve. I want you to have a vision for your life. Once you understand what the finished product (your life) can look like by implementing this plan, I believe you will become a powerful force of positive energy. Seeing what your life could look like and knowing that these benefits await you will inspire you to take action. Let's talk about the benefits of this plan and what it will help you create. Consider this plan the design and know that you are the engineer who is putting it together step by step.

You'll Have More Energy

One of the most common statements I hear from people about this plan is that they feel "much more energized, alive, and awake." It's as if this plan represents a flashlight that helps take us through the darkness and clutter of stress, fatigue, and to-do lists to find our energy switch. By implementing this plan, we are in essence turning on this energy switch, and the more we turn it on the stronger and more prevalent this energy becomes. Each 10-minute exercise represents the turning on of our energy switch, and the result is more energy for our lives and careers. Energy begets energy, and by focusing your energy on increasing your energy, you grow your energy. This plan also gives you more energy because it includes various exercises that increase all your sources of energy. This creates an upward energy spiral effect where the physical exercise boosts your mental and emotional energy, and the mental/emotional exercise boosts your physical energy. Physical activity impacts our thoughts and emotions, and our thoughts and emotions affect us physically. Our physical, mental, and emotional energy is all spiraled together, and by energizing each component as part of a complete plan, you gain significant benefits. But don't take my word for it. Try this energy experiment for yourself and see how good you feel. Like anything, what you put into it is what you will get out of it. So make sure you take action, invest your energy, and let this plan pay you big energy returns.

You'll Increase Your Happiness

> "A man is about as happy as he chooses to be."
> —Abraham Lincoln

With all this stress in your life and the negativity in the world, you may wonder at times if there's any hope. "What's the point?" you may ask. You may feel so overwhelmed you don't know where to begin.

When I feel like this, I think of a story I once heard about a man who goes to the village to speak to the wise man. He is granted a question to ask the wise man and he says, "I feel like there are two dogs inside me. One dog is this positive loving, kind, gentle, and happy dog. The other dog is this mean, angry, negative, and sad dog. And they fight all the time. I don't know what to do. I don't know who is going to win." After contemplating this quandary for a moment, the wise man answers, "I know who is going to win. The one you feed the most. So feed the positive dog."

This is the choice we have every moment of every day. We can feed the negativity in our life, or we can feed the positive energy. We can fuel the darkness or turn on the light. This plan will help us go on a negative energy starvation diet and nourish ourselves with positive energy. This plan represents the food we need to feed our positive dog, and the more we feed this dog the bigger it will grow.

We have the opportunity every moment of every day to create our own happiness. You can create the life you want one thought, one word, one belief, one choice, one action at a time. This isn't just a theory or hokey self-improvement mumbo jumbo. It's neuroscience. Daniel Goleman's incredible book *Destructive Emotions* explains the latest research in neuroscience, and the picture this research paints is that for humans, finding our "light switch" and "feeding the positive dog" means activating the part of our brain associated with happy feelings and positive emotions.

According to Richard Davidson, professor of psychology and psychiatry at the University of Wisconsin in Madison, people who have high levels of brain activity in the left prefrontal cortex experience feelings such as happiness, enthusiasm, joy, high energy, and alertness. But people with a high level of activity in the right prefrontal cortex are more prone to feelings of sadness, anxiety, and worry. According to Davidson, we each have a characteristic ration of left to right activation that offers a barometer of the moods we are likely to feel each day. He calls this a leftward tilt (positive emotions) or rightward tilt (negative emotions). This can also be called a "happiness set point" that neuroscience experts believe we are born with.

David Lykken, a University of Minnesota psychology professor, has found through his research on twins that there is amazingly little connection between one's life circumstance and one's predominant moods. Even lottery winners and paraplegics return to their usual temperament within a year of their winning or accident. While events and circumstances such as winning the lottery, finding a new job, falling in love, or receiving a promotion may make you happier in the short run, over time you will return to your usual happiness set point. However, research by Davidson and others also shows that our brain is plastic and can be molded by repetitive experience and repetitive activity. Think of yourself with a happiness meter or thermostat inside you. Now realize that this happiness thermostat can be changed only from the inside, not the outside. External events won't do it. The happiness set point can be moved only from the inside and the goal is to move it to the left. Davidson's research shows that we can create a tilt toward our left prefrontal cortex and enlarge and strengthen certain areas of the brain by repetitively and habitually using and exercising those areas. In other words, we can "learn" to be happy. Consider the following studies.

➤ A study by Edward Taub, a behavioral neuroscientist at the University of Alabama, Birmingham, and Thomas Elbert of the University of Konstanz, Germany, shows that trained musicians enlarge relevant parts of the brain. Hours and hours on the violin change the amount of cells involved in musical performance, enhance their conductivity, and rewire the brain.

➤ A study on London taxicab drivers that was published in *Nature* stated that the areas of the brain associated with navigation and direction were strengthened after the first six months of driving their taxis around the streets of London.

➤ Research by Richard Davidson, Ph.D., at the University of Wisconsin demonstrates that regular meditation increases activation in the left prefrontal cortex. This activity is associated with lower anxiety, a more positive emotional state, and better immune system function, according to the study.

Now, think about a skill that you use in your work or life. Now think about how accomplished you were at this skill when you first started. Whether it's making lunch for the kids, making sales calls, or learning how to type, it was awkward at first. But over time, after much practice, it became second nature. Now you don't even have to think about it. It's become automatic. It becomes a habit. Our brain responds to our actions and our actions respond to our brain.

Positive and negative thinking works the same way. So while each of us may be born with a certain happiness set point or mood barometer, neuroscience research tells us it can be shifted and changed by cultivating repetitive thoughts, experiences, and emotions that consistently activate the left prefrontal cortex. The more we do this, the more automatic this response becomes and the more this area of the brain is strengthened. Like feeding the positive dog, this is what grows. We can actually rewire our brains to create more activation in our left prefrontal cortex, or in regard to our happiness set point, we move our energy thermostat to the left.

Happiness and positive energy, then, are not things that happen to us, like a lightning strike, but rather something that we create. This is a skill that can be acquired. It is a habit. Just as practicing hitting a golf ball will make you a better golfer or taking piano lessons will make you a better pianist, practicing skills that cultivate happiness will make you happier. While you may have been born with a negative temperament or cultivated a negative mind-set by habitual negative thinking, you have the power to change. We are all born with certain skill levels; some are happier, better singers, piano players, artists, and athletes. Yet with practice we can all grow and improve our skill. So, no matter what your happiness set point may be now, know that with dedication and practice, you can move it to the left.

You can mold your brain to become more positive. Einstein referred to certain mental experiences as "muscular," and like any physical muscle we can build our mental, emotional, and spiritual muscles to make them stronger, more positive, more resistant to stress, and more active. Just as lifting weights on a regular basis builds physical muscles, we can practice specific mental and emotional exercises to build mental and emotional muscle. We can build more happiness instead of sadness. More trust instead of fear. More calm instead of stress. More positive energy instead of negative energy. And the best part about building mental and emotional muscle is that it doesn't take a lot of time. Repetition is the key and 10 minutes a day is all it takes to produce lifelong results.

You'll Learn to Trust Yourself

"Trust your hopes, not your fears."

—David Mahoney

Trust is the antidote to fear. Trust helps replace fearful thoughts that say, "Everything bad always happens to me," with a belief that

"Everything happens for a reason." Whereas fear creates struggle, trust creates peace. Whereas fear seeks to separate, trust unites. Fear causes anxiety, unhappiness, and stress, but trust creates peace, calm, and happiness. The 10-Minute-a-Day Plan helps you create more trust and less fear in your life. It helps you build the trust you'll need to overcome and override the fear that can run rampant through your life. This plan helps you develop the mental and emotional strength you'll need to turn off the faucet of fear and prevent fear energy from overflowing and drowning you in misery. No longer will you serve your fear. Rather, your fear will serve you. The power of building trust becomes evident when you understand how trust and fear tango inside the three parts of our brain.

Neurologist Paul MacLean developed the model that humans actually have "three brains in one" that interact like three interconnected computers. He classified the three parts of the brain according to evolutionary development. MacLean calls the lower part of the brain the reptilian brain. It includes the brain stem and the cerebellum. The reptilian part of the brain, like a lizard, is all about instinct and survival. There's no emotion whatsoever—this is why alligators will never replace dogs as the family pet! The reptilian brain controls digestion, reproduction, circulation, breathing, and the execution of the fight-or-flight response. It is all about fear, survival, and dominance.

The second part of the brain is the limbic system, your brain's emotional center, which houses the amygdala. The amygdala is your "warehouse of fear." It remembers everything that could cause you hurt or pain. The amygdala reminds you to look left and right twice before crossing the street so you don't get hit by a car. My amygdala is what causes me to use the chain lock to secure my hotel door, since I didn't use it one time and someone broke in to my room while I was sleeping. Ever since then, my amygdala reminds me to double lock my door.

The amygdala also makes judgments. It decides good or bad. Pleasure or pain. From a survival standpoint, it makes sense that the amygdala is connected to the fight-or-flight fear response system that pumps stress hormones through you when you are feeling fearful or anxious. Instead of rationalizing whether something was going to eat you or not, your amygdala would make an immediate judgment and kick into gear and your emotional fearful response would get you moving quickly to safety. Who has time to think when a tiger is about to eat you? We need an immediate response system for survival, and we've got it.

The third and higher part of the brain is called the neocortex, and it constitutes five-sixths of our brain. MacLean believes it was the last part of our brain to evolve; it is what separates humans from animals. The neocortex gives us the ability to think, rationalize, and trust, and it is the site of creativity, intuition, compassion, and intelligence. When you think, you use your neocortex. When you pray or have an intellectual conversation, you use your neocortex.

There is ongoing communication among the three brains via a network of neurons, nerves, and electrical pathways that link thinking, emotions, and actions. While the reptilian brain and the limbic system coordinate to remember and act upon a fearful event, the neocortex and the limbic system via its vast network of neurological connections work together to think, feel, trust, and love.

How we think, feel, act, and live, then, is a function of which part of the brain is in charge and how our three brains are interacting. If you are someone who is in a constant state of fear, then you have an overactive reptilian brain and amygdala, and you are underutilizing your neocortex. In fact, research by Richard Davidson shows that amygdalas are more active in people who are depressed. On the other hand, if you are someone who can stay calm during a crisis, you have obviously learned to effectively use your neocortex to override your primitive fear response system. We all know people who tend to over-rationalize and overanalyze, which leads to "paralysis by analysis." These people are often looked at as being apathetic or emotionless. On the other hand, we all know people who are impulsive. They likely have not learned to rationalize and utilize their neocortex. Like children, they grab what they want. They lead a fear-based existence.

The purpose of the 10-Minute-a-Day Plan, then, is to help you learn to override your reptilian brain and negative emotions with your higher brain, positive emotions, and positive energy that serve you. When you think about it, this is an amazing revelation. By learning to trust and use our higher brain more, we can override and overcome our fear. We can stop it from hijacking our brain and thought process. We can tell ourselves, "It's going to be okay" . . . "calm down . . . trust." Instead of letting our lower brain influence our higher brain, we can train the higher brain to influence the lower brain. We can tame and train our reptilian brain. Like a parent talking to a child, we can teach it to stop overreacting and causing so much trouble. When our boss gives us a dirty look, instead of going into survival mode, we can trust that everything will work out. When dealing with a traumatic event in our life, we can trust and hope in the future. If we are having a conflict with a coworker or relative, we can trust that it is presenting us with a lesson.

Most often, the first response to any difficult situation will be fear. It's the way we were designed. However, since we are blessed with the neocortex, we have the ability to think, trust, and pray to overcome this instinctual fear. And I have found (and so have thousands of others) that the more we do the exercises in this book, the more we are able to overcome the fear that used to sabotage our health, happiness, career, and relationships. By consistently and constantly choosing trust and prayer to override fear, we decrease the power and influence of the reptilian brain over our thinking process.

The ultimate choice we have every moment of every day is to trust or to fear. This plan is designed to help you choose trust. When you trust, instead of trying to survive, you'll learn to thrive. Instead of struggling through life, you'll learn to flow. And instead of always fearing the worst, you'll learn to trust and hope for the best. Trust will replace fear. Hope will replace hopelessness. Optimism will replace pessimism. And surrender will replace your need for control. Although fear energy may serve you temporarily, it eventually runs out. Trust, however, is high-octane fuel for the journey of life. It will take you where you are supposed to go—if you let it.

You'll Increase Your Emotional Energy

> "Emotions are like fire. They can cook your food and keep you warm or they can burn your house down."
> —Cus D'Amato, the boxing trainer who taught Mike Tyson

If you followed the career and life of Mike Tyson, you know he burned down his house many times. Emotions are extremely powerful forces of charged energy, and they can ignite us to act positively or negatively. If you have ever been in a bad mood or felt in a funk for no apparent reason, you know how negative emotions can create an intense charge of negative energy that causes a downward spiral of sadness, fatigue, apathy, and depression. On the other hand, if you have ever been at a party feeling bored and someone brings up a topic that you absolutely love, you know how positive emotions can wake you up and make you feel alive. If you have ever been in a packed football stadium during a big game, you understand the electricity that is produced by a collection of emotionally charged people. And if you have ever been at a family gathering where two relatives get into a fight, you know how negative emotions and negative energy can create tension so thick you could almost cut it with a knife!

Emotions are electrifying, and they have the ability to help us create success or failure, happiness or sadness, and abundance or scarcity. The purpose of the 10-Minute-a-Day Plan is to help you cultivate more positive emotions in your life. While research shows that our mood and thoughts affect emotions, which in turn affect our physiology, we also know that we can positively charge our emotions to change our mood and thoughts. If you have ever had to put your game face on for an important meeting or sports event, or you've mentally prepared yourself before a family gathering, you know what it's like to take control of your emotions.

By charging our emotions in a positive way, we can stop the downward cycle of despair in its tracks. Instead of allowing our emotions to dictate how we think and feel, we can take control of emotions, thoughts, and feelings. While some may call this a "fake until you make it" approach, I call it building mental and emotional muscle. When you cultivate specific emotions you want to experience, and you train yourself to charge up with these emotions, you'll create an optimal state of mind and body. At first, charging your emotions will feel awkward. But like riding a bike or wearing a watch on your opposite hand, over time it will become natural. Like eating, thinking, and drinking, emotions are a habit. The positive emotions you cultivate while doing this plan will become a part of you, and this will positively impact every area of your life.

You'll Reduce Your Stress

> "While we may not be able to control all that happens to us, we can control what happens inside us."
> —Benjamin Franklin

The age of physical strength is over. Darwin's "survival of the fittest" is history. Unless you are a soldier or living in the wilderness, rarely does one have to run from a tiger or fight hand-to-hand combat anymore. Survival today depends much less on our physical ability to conquer someone and much more on our ability to transform and manage stress. Consider that more than half of all deaths between the ages of one and sixty-five result from stressful lifestyles, according to the Centers for Disease Control.

In our energy-strapped, technology-driven, time-constrained society, the new law of the land is survival of the calmest. I call it "Conscious Darwinism." Instead of evolving physically to meet the attacks of predators, we must evolve consciously to meet the challenges of a radically changing society. After all, it's not the tigers and wild animals but our own fearful, stressful, and negative thoughts that cause us harm. Instead of fighting other tribes, now we must fight the lines at Starbucks and battle traffic during our daily commutes. Everywhere you turn people are stressed out.

Conscious Darwinism is not such a radical thought when you realize, as I mentioned before, that over 90 percent of doctor visits are due to stress-related causes. Think of stress as a dam or wall that blocks a flowing river, causing stagnant water and the buildup of toxins, bacteria, pesticides, and other harmful influences. In our flowing, energetic bodies, stress creates an energy blockage that stops the healthy flow of our energetic system. Since energy creates matter, energy blockages create physical blocks. It's no surprise then that stress has been linked to hardening of the arteries and less blood flow to the heart. Our energetic reality determines our physical reality. When our energy is stagnant, we are more prone to toxins and illnesses.

Since stress is taking such a toll on our health and society, reducing stress is the most essential survival strategy we all need now. Those who learn to transform their stress will not only survive but also thrive. We must evolve consciously and learn to become calm in the midst of turmoil. We must learn to take on each day with thoughts, strategies, and techniques that help us flow through life instead of fighting each day. I know it's not easy, but for those who want to maintain their health and energy, it is essential. Thankfully, this plan will help you do just that. You'll reduce your stress, evolve consciously, and make better choices that will help you live a longer, calmer, and healthier life.

You'll Let Go of Negativity

> "For every minute you are angry you lose
> sixty seconds of happiness."
>
> —Ralph Waldo Emerson

One of the most important discoveries I made while coaching people is that no matter how much you try to charge yourself up with positive emotion, thoughts, and affirmations, you'll still feel stuck if you don't let go of the negativity that holds you back. I realized this after I saw all these people do all these great exercises and create incredible belief systems and take serious action steps . . . and yet they still failed to create the results they desired. I realized that we are like an energy pipeline, and no matter how much we charge up with positive energy, it doesn't work if there is too much sludge inside us. As in any healthy ecosystem, the removal of waste and toxins is important to the overall health of the system. Every aspect of our lives involves waste removal so that the energy can flow. Garbage is removed from our houses, toxins and metabolic by-products are removed from our bodies, and poisonous influences are removed from a farmer's land. Like everything in nature, we need to remove the mental and emotional toxins that prevent us from growing and building muscle. We must remove the sludge inside our energy pipeline. Not doing so would be like letting the garbage pile up on the side of our house. We must let go so we can flow.

This "negative sludge" comes in the form of anger, resentment, self-doubt, past painful events, emotional pain, and fear. Negative emotions and thought patterns occupy your energy field with heavy lower-vibration energy that actually weighs you down physically, mentally, emotionally, and spiritually. No matter how much you try to fill up with positive energy, if you have this junk within you, the positive energy cannot flow through. This sludge holds you back, causes resistance and disharmony in your body, and manifests itself as an unfulfilled life and unrealized potential. This heavy energy stops the flow of abundant energy in your life and will likely cause you to ask, "Why am I not happy and why is my life not going the way I thought it would?" I know because I used to ask these questions all the time. Only when I let go of the fear, resistance, and emotional pain that was holding me back did my life start flowing abundantly.

If you have ever forgiven someone and felt as if a weight has been lifted off your life, you know how heavy this sludge can be. If you have ever rid yourself of a bad relationship and felt one hundred pounds lighter and freer, you know how your emotions can affect you mentally and physically. We all have sludge inside us. Not a pretty picture, but it's true. It is part of the human experience. Many of the people I coach have been abused, forgotten, ignored, and abandoned. They hold on to these painful events and feelings without realizing it, and they never make the connection between their emotional pain and their low energy and unhappiness. Once they understand this connection, let go of their emotional pain, and start doing the exercises I'm going to share with you in this book, everything changes. Their energy shifts and their life improves. They feel lighter, freer, and happier, and so will you.

You'll Find Silence

> "True silence is the rest of the mind, and is to the spirit what sleep is to the body, nourishment and refreshment."
>
> —William Penn

The power of silence is available to all of us, but unfortunately in today's noisy world filled with cars, sirens, telephone rings, video games, and television, silence is undervalued and underutilized. Even when we have time for silence, we opt to pick up our cell phone and make a call instead. Rarely do we just sit still to hear the sound of our breath and feel the beat of our heart and connect with the stillness of our soul. Within every moment of silence is a powerful source of silent energy that can recharge your mind, energize your body, and refuel your life. Silent energy is potential energy. Before the booming sound of thunder, there is silence. Before an orchestra plays beautiful music, there is silence. Before a powerful hit on a baseball field, there is silence. Everything is born out of silence. Silent energy is infinite energy. When you find time for silence, you tap into a boundless source of energy that birthed the sun, moon, and stars. This silence is all around you and the goal in life is to tap it.

This plan will help you create moments of silence and tap silent energy. Instead of always filling your life with business and noise, you will find brief moments of stillness and silence. Instead of always using and expending energy like a NASCAR race car, this plan will help you take times throughout your day to make a pit stop and fuel up at the "silent energy" gas station. You'll realize what the best race car drivers already know. You can't keep expending energy without making the time to stop and refuel. Those who ignore their energy needs run out of gas and blow out their engine. When you find silence with this plan, you will find an energy source that is always available to you. You won't have to drive to a gas station. You'll be able to stop, find a brief moment of silence, and fill up anytime and anywhere.

You'll Feel the Flow

> "If you wish to glimpse inside a human soul, just
> watch a person laugh and play. Those who laugh
> and play well are the most alive."
>
> —Fyodor Dostoyevsky

"Flow," a term coined by University of Chicago psychologist Mihaly Csikszentmihalyi refers to an optimal experience or feeling of being engaged with life. I like to think of flow as an experience of your energy field becoming one with the energy that is all around you. This happens when you are in the present moment. It happens when you are doing something you love—something meaningful, something fun. Flow happens when you are playing, when you are in pursuit of a meaningful goal, or as many of us have experienced when we are playing sports, meditating, laughing with friends, or sometimes just walking along the beach. Instead of thinking about your problems, issues, and challenges, you are not thinking at all. You are just being. When this happens, your energy changes. It's as if you literally become lighter, bouncier, and freer, and I believe future research will show that during times of flow we experience an energy frequency change at the cellular and energy level. We are energy beings and when our energy changes, we change. But we don't have to wait for future research to experience the benefits of flow. This plan will help you get engaged with life and feel the flow. You'll be reminded of what it feels like to have fun. You'll experience more smiles, more laughs, and more moments of silence. You'll feel more connected to yourself, to others, and to your higher power. And you'll become one with the present moment and with life itself. Instead of fighting life, you will flow with it.

You'll Develop Spiritual Muscle and Create Miracles

> "As for me, I know nothing else but miracles."
> —Walt Whitman

Like happiness, spiritual muscle is not something that just happens to us. It is created through our thoughts, words, and belief system.

Einstein said, "There are only two ways to live your life. One is as though nothing is a miracle. The other is as though everything is a miracle." When you believe everything is a miracle, you see little miracles all around you. As if you had put on a new pair of glasses, the world looks different. You see the miracle of life in a newborn baby. You feel the miracle of love in a warm embrace. You observe the miracle of a greater intelligence inside you. After all, when you eat, do you worry about digesting the food and distributing the nutrients to your cells and eliminating the toxins that could make you ill? No, you eat and you let your miraculous design do the rest.

When you develop spiritual muscle, you marvel at the miracle of the grand design in something as small and seemingly insignificant as an apple seed. For inside this one seed is the potential for an apple tree that produces bunches of apples that contain more seeds that grow more trees that grow more apples. Insignificance turns to awe when you realize that within one seed is the potential for an infinite supply of apples. The miracle becomes clear. The same abundance we see in an apple seed is also inside you and all around you. Miracles are not in short supply. They are abundant too. We just have to plant the seeds that grow miracles. These seeds come in the form of our thoughts, and they develop and grow with a miracle mind-set. And the more we practice a miracle mind-set the more spiritual muscle we create.

When you have a miracle mind-set, you believe that everything is a miracle—you perceive miracles all around you, you expect miracles to happen in every day of your life, you look for miracles and wait for them to happen—but you don't attach to them. Instead, you wait with awe and know that miracles happen in God's time, not your time.

Consider two people on a roller coaster. One is terrified and the other is laughing and having the time of her life. They get off the ride, and one feels sick, while the other feels exuberant. Two different people with two different perceptions produce two very different experiences and realities. Clearly, the world we see and experience is defined by the lenses through which we observe it. So when you create a miracle mind-set that thinks about, prays for, and expects miracles, you place your energy and attention on miracles. Just as when you buy a new car and start to notice that car everywhere, when you focus your attention on miracles, you start to see and experience them more in your life. The more you create a miracle mind-set and wear your miracle glasses the more automatic this way of thinking becomes. It becomes a habit, and this helps you build spiritual muscle.

So in the 10-Minute-a-Day Plan I will help you create a miracle mind-set that helps you build spiritual muscle. When faced with life's struggles, spiritual muscle will help you shift your ordinary mind-set to a miracle mind-set. Instead of seeing the problem, you'll see the lesson. Instead of seeing the crisis, you'll see the opportunity. Conflicts will become lessons. Pain will become part of growth. Obstacles will become hurdles to success and paths to a better you. As you build spiritual muscle, you'll be able to respond to life's challenges and crises with more calm, more peace, and more understanding. Sure you will still feel pain. You are human. But you'll be in touch with a greater and higher source of energy to help you handle and overcome this pain. Instead of becoming an emotional basket case, you will be a powerful force of love, trust, and spiritual strength.

You'll Create Coherence in Your Life

What is "coherence" in terms of energy? Coherence has to do with the heart's electromagnetic field and how it impacts your energy mentally, physically, and emotionally. The latest research in neurocardiology by the Institute of HeartMath (www.heartmath.org) demonstrates that:

1. The heart's electromagnetic field is five thousand times more powerful than the brain.
2. The heart is more than a mechanical blood pump; it is a dynamic and intelligent sensory organ that plays the role of emotional conductor in your body and influences how you think and feel.
3. Electromagnetic waves identifying a person's emotional state are communicated throughout the body via the heart's electromagnetic field, and the rhythmic beating patterns of the heart change significantly as a person experiences different emotions.
4. Negative emotions such as anger, jealousy, or frustration are associated with erratic, disordered, incoherent patterns in the heart rhythms.
5. Positive emotions such as love, compassion, and appreciation are associated with a smooth, ordered, coherent pattern in the heart's rhythmic activity.
6. Coherence and incoherence influence the structure of the electromagnetic field radiated by the heart to every cell in the body.
7. Coherence leads to an organized electromagnetic field, which enhances health and well-being.

So what does all this mean to you and me? Simply put, our emotions influence how our heart interacts with our body and brain. Imagine that the heart is like the conductor of an orchestra. Each cell in our body is like a musical instrument. When the conductor experiences happy and positive emotions, he is coherent and improves communication between the instruments and with the instruments. Each instrument is in tune with the other, even though they all may all be playing different notes. Communication is enhanced and everything is synchronized magically. The result is beautiful music. On the other hand, when the conductor is angry and upset, he doesn't perform as well. He is incoherent. Communication is poor. The instruments become out of sync and the music is awful.

In our lives the heart plays the role of conductor. When it feels good, you feel good. The body is in a state of harmony. Cell to cell communication improves and flows. Stress is reduced, health is enhanced, performance increases, intuitional insight becomes more common, and mental clarity increases. Beautiful music in our orchestra analogy correlates to physical, mental, and emotional health, increased energy, and happiness.

The goal of the 10-Minute-a-Day Plan, then, is to help you create sustained positive emotions that will help you create coherence and enhance the functioning and power of your heart's electromagnetic field. In turn, you will broadcast a powerful and positive message to your mind and body and achieve an optimal state of mental, physical, and emotional health. You will create heartfelt emotions that radiate love, trust, abundance, joy, and compassion to every cell in your body and every ounce of your consciousness. This will improve the way you think about life, the way you feel about yourself, and the energy you project to the world.

Now that you have a vision for what you can create with this plan, I hope this inspires you even more to put the 10-Minute-a-Day Plan into action. I believe this plan will help you turn this vision into your life. Everything you just read is possible if you are willing to take action. With the thousands of people I have coached, I have found that the talkers talk and the doers do. Now, I hope you are ready to be a doer. In the next chapter I'll explain how the 10-Minute Energy Solution works, and then you'll be ready to take action.

Chapter 4

Putting the Plan into Action

The Anti–Quick Fix Program

This is not a quick fix program. While the 10-Minute Energy Solution may sound like some six-pack abdominal muscle commercial, I want to be very clear that there's no magic pill or special gizmo here to get you to your goals. This program is intended to impact the rest of your life; it's a lifestyle change, not a quick fix. In fact, I believe this is the *anti*–quick fix program needed in today's quick fix culture.

But at the same time, the program isn't complicated, and it doesn't take up your entire life. That's the beauty of 10 Minutes a Day. Let's face it, people are busy. We're all looking for help, but if a plan is complicated, confusing, and long, we are probably not going to stick with it. With so many quick fixes available to us 24/7, I felt the need to create a solution that countered the quick fix culture and showed hardworking people that if they make small, simple, effortless changes in their daily routine, they will produce powerful, lasting results.

Can I Really Change *Anything* in 10 Minutes a Day?

Life is all about the little things. It's one of my central philosophies that has helped thousands of people produce results. Sometimes people mock my approach because it seems too easy and obvious. They might say, "You're not telling me anything new." Some people wonder if this 10-Minute-a-Day program really is so easy, why aren't more people doing it? I tell them that so many of us overlook the little things because they happen to be right in front of our faces.

We may all know what we need to do, but we don't do it. We get so busy that we forget to do the basics. Then, when we get lost, we start looking for the holy grail of a solution, thinking it has to be a long, complicated quest. Then when someone like me comes along, gives you a plan, and says, "Hey you should try this," it reminds you of what you already know but forgot. So you do the little things, and they make you feel great. Then, since you feel great, you do them again and again—producing amazing results. You are truly surprised that the little things had such an impact on your life, but you can't dispute how you feel. You become a believer. You realize that the amazing results—happiness, energy, contentment—were always just one small step away from you. You just had to take that step to discover it.

How the Plan Works

10 Minutes a Day for Thirty Days

➤   Each day for thirty days I will share with you a 10-minute exercise. I will explain to you the purpose of this exercise, why it works, and how to do it.

➤ Each week, the 10-minute exercises will focus on a specific theme. For example, one week we'll focus on adding 10 minutes of positive action to each day; during another week we'll focus on losing 10 minutes of negative energy in your day.

➤ You'll want to review each day's exercise the night before so you can plan for it.

➤ You will then schedule this exercise in your calendar, planner, PDA, or whatever method you use to plan your day.

➤ If you schedule your 10-minute exercise, you are more likely to do it.

➤ By the end of the day, you will complete your 10-minute exercise.

➤ Each one of the 10-minute exercises will guide your actions and help you produce results. Just as singers perform vocal exercises to strengthen their voices, we must do exercises for our mind that build mental, emotional, and spiritual muscle. And just as different weight-lifting exercises build different physical muscles in your body, you'll find that these 10-minute exercises build different mental, emotional, and spiritual muscles. Each exercise has a purpose and is designed to achieve a desired result.

Note

While the plan calls for you to do only one 10-minute exercise a day, if you really fall in love with one or more of the exercises and you want to keep on doing them on other days, then simply add this exercise to the exercise I have presented to you on that day. It's not required, but when people have done this plan in the past, I had many inquiries to do more than one exercise a day. I certainly don't want to hold you back. If something works and you want to keep on doing it, then I encourage you wholeheartedly. For example, when you do the thank-you walk on the first day and you decide that you want to also do it on the second day, then simply do the exercise for day 2 and then do the thank-you walk as well. I have found that with just 10 minutes a day you will see great results, but if you want to achieve even more results, then I say go for it.

The 11th-Minute Miracle

If you're someone who wants to build spiritual muscle also, I have included a one-minute prayer exercise that will follow each daily 10-minute exercise. I call it the 11th-Minute Miracle because devoting even just one minute a day to your higher power will help you create more miracles in your life—starting with the miracle of health and happiness.

Studies have shown a connection between spirituality, health, and happiness and even one minute a day will help you create this connection and reap the benefits. According to David Meyers, author of *The Pursuit of Happiness,* study after study shows that highly religious and spiritual people are happier and they cope better with crisis. Paramahansa Yogananda wrote, "God is the repository of all happiness; and you can contact him in everyday life. Yet man mostly occupies himself in pursuits that lead to unhappiness."

The 11th-Minute Miracle is meant to help you take the time to make this important connection and discover the happiness you seek. I have found that if you just start with a minute, that one minute spreads beyond, impacting your entire day and your life. You'll love it so much that you'll get addicted to it in a positive way. In my own life I have found prayer to be a powerful source of energy. I believe it will also provide you with life-changing fuel. Einstein said, "We cannot solve our problems with the same thinking we used when we created them." The 11th-Minute Miracle represents a higher level of thinking that will provide us with the solutions to our daily struggles and challenges. If something hasn't been working in your life, a new approach is needed and the 11th-Minute Miracle is one such approach.

Note

Although I use the term God, I encourage you to use the term that feels most comfortable to you. I am not here to convince you to believe in a certain religion but rather to help you connect to your higher power and feel a spiritual connection with the divine source and ultimate fuel for your life. Each person has a plan and a path, and I trust you will find your own way. My hope is that this plan, like a compass, helps you find your direction.

Note

While I wrote a specific 11th-Minute Miracle after each 10-minute exercise, I encourage you to say your own prayers if you are more comfortable with them or say one of the following three prayers instead.

Prayer of St. Francis

Lord, make me an instrument of Your peace.

Where there is hatred, let me sow love;

where there is injury, pardon;

where there is doubt, faith;

where there is despair, hope;

where there is darkness, light;

and where there is sadness, joy.

O, Divine Master,

grant that I may not so much seek

to be consoled as to console;

to be understood as to understand;

to be loved as to love;

for it is in giving that we receive;

it is in pardoning that we are pardoned;

and it is in dying that we are born to eternal life.

The Serenity Prayer

God grant me the serenity to accept the things I cannot change, courage to change the things I can, and wisdom to know the difference.

—Reinhold Niebuhr

When I Let Go and Let God

Doors fly open, Gates lift, Attitudes shift

Paths clear, Ways appear

Obstacles dissolve, Mountains move

Traffic parts, Green lights shine

Red carpets roll out, Abundance rolls in

Opportunity Knocks, Life rocks

Well-being abounds

I let it in!

Grateful I am!

—Judee Pouncey

Track Your Energy Foundation

I also include the following progress tracker for you to complete at the end of each day. This tracker will help you hold yourself accountable as you create your essential energy foundation. You will simply check off each habit that you implemented that day.

I ate breakfast.	■
I ate smaller healthy meals and energizing snacks.	■
I drank plenty of water.	■
I slept enough to feel energized and rested.	■
I engaged in some form of physical activity.	■

I listened to energizing music.	■
I connected with people who increase my energy.	■
I practiced my energizer breath when stressed.	■

Energy Scales

I also provide you with several scales to help you measure where you are at each point of the plan. Using the scales below, you'll establish a starting point. These scales are subjective because the only thing that matters is how you feel about your life. These scales are a simple way for you to check in with yourself and your progress. As you follow the plan, I will present the scales to you after the seventh, fourteenth, twenty-first, twenty-eighth, and thirtieth day for you to measure yourself. I will also ask you a few questions that will help you further measure your progress. Establish your starting point using the scales below.

Negative Energy–Positive Energy Scale

1	2	3	4	5	6	7	8	9	10

Negative   Positive

To help you pick a number that applies to you, consider this framework.

1—You embody pessimism to the degree that not only do you see the glass as half empty but don't even like the glass. You are very negative and very rarely see the good in anyone or anything.

10—You are an optimist who is positively energized by people and life itself. People always comment on your positive energy.

Sad-Happy Scale

1	2	3	4	5	6	7	8	9	10

Sad   Happy

To help you pick a number that applies to you, consider this framework.

1—You feel miserable, unhappy, depressed, and sad. You often feel hopeless.

10—You feel happy and content with your life. You feel like the happiest person on earth.

Stressed Scale

1	2	3	4	5	6	7	8	9	10

Stressed   Relaxed

To help you pick a number that applies to you, consider this framework.

1—You feel overwhelmed, stressed, and at any moment you could lose it. You can't breathe and you think about all you have to do instead of enjoying life.

10—You stay completely calm and know that everything will get done as it always does. You are the calm in the midst of turmoil. Everyone comments on how calm you always are.

Focused Scale

1	2	3	4	5	6	7	8	9	10

Scattered   Focused

To help you pick a number that applies to you, consider this framework.

1—You are all over the place. You feel like your energy is in five places at once. You can't concentrate and you feel that your life is spinning. You feel like a juggler who does a million things but can't focus and enjoy one of them. Your energy feels scattered and weak.

10—Like a laser, you feel very focused and you focus on one thing at a time. Your energy feels centered and powerful.

Fear-Trust Scale

1	2	3	4	5	6	7	8	9	10

Fear   Trust

To help you pick a number on the scale that applies to you, consider this framework.

1—You feel worried, anxious, and fearful all the time. Fear consumes you.

10—You look at problems and challenges as paths to growth, and you trust that great things are happening.

Overall Energy Scale

1	2	3	4	5	6	7	8	9	10

Low   High

To help you pick a number on the scale that applies to you, consider this framework.

1—You can't even get out of bed. You are drained. Your energy meter is on 0.

10—You are completely energized. Your energy meter is full, and you don't think it could go any higher.

Tools for Success

As an Energy Coach, I have come to realize the profound reality that change is not always easy—even if you make it as easy as possible with a 10-minutes-a-day approach. People often fail at plans and diets because changes are not easy to maintain. New habits often feel awkward.

Habits take time to develop, and in order for them to produce lasting results I believe habits and plans need to stick to your life. They have to become a part of you. But, unfortunately, when you are trying new habits and engaging in new behaviors, a number of obstacles appear. These obstacles often cause you to give up before these positive and powerful habits have the opportunity to become a natural part of your life. These obstacles might include missing a day of the plan, feeling like a failure, self-doubt, lack of motivation, lack of support, or hopelessness.

I have found through my coaching that if people can overcome these obstacles and get over the hump, they can make significant long-lasting changes. This is accomplished by incorporating resources, tools, and support that will help you create success. You understand the roadblocks before they even start, which is why we are talking about this before you start the plan. And you have a solution before the problem even arises. So before you start the plan, I want to offer you a few tools for success that will help you overcome the obstacles I have seen occur for many people just like you.

1. **Team up.** If you are someone who has trouble sticking to plans by yourself but are energized by others, find a friend, coworker,

or family member to do this plan with you. Become accountability partners and help each other stick to the plan. We see the concept of teamwork in fire departments, police stations, and sports teams all the time, and this same approach is possible for our lives when we are doing this plan.

2. **Find a coach or counselor.** Even the best athletes need coaches. We all need help in staying focused, disciplined, and inspired. Although we *can* do it alone, there are times when a coach makes all the difference. If you know you are someone who needs a coach or mentor, then don't feel ashamed—you are not alone. Success is never created in a vacuum but rather with the love, support, and help of others. Coaches give us a hug when we need some support and a kick in the rear when we need a little push in the right direction. Coaches also can help hold you accountable while sharing the positive energy and enthusiasm you need to keep you inspired.

    The power of having a coach was clear during my appearances on the NBC *Today* show, where I coached three women to increase their energy over thirty days. I believe one of the reasons why the three women I coached achieved such dramatic results was because I called them every day. Energy is contagious, and my energy inspired them to take action. Now I'm not saying that you need a coach to make this plan a success. My goal with this plan was to be your coach in book form. However, if you believe that having the guidance, support, and inspiration of a live coach will help you make long-lasting changes, then I say go for it. Feel free to e-mail me and I can refer you to an energy coach I have personally trained. Or take this plan to your life coach or therapist, and ask him to coach you through this plan.

3. **Sign up for my free weekly newsletter.** It provides you with a weekly reminder to focus on your health, happiness, and positive

energy. As I have often heard from people, it energizes you more than a shot of espresso. It will help you stay energized and on track. Most of all, my goal each week is to offer a ray of hope when you need it most. To sign up for my free newsletter, visit www.jongordon.com.

4. **Visit my website and listen to my weekly encouragements.** I have set up a special page on my website (www.jongordon.com) for people who are following this plan. On this page I have included weekly encouragements to help you through common challenges and roadblocks. I have also included other tools for success, so visit this website at your convenience if you need help, support, and guidance.

5. **Don't let one or two days ruin a plan for the rest of your life.** If something comes up in your life and you happen to miss a day or even a few days of this plan, don't stop. Instead of giving up, use this time to pause. Missing one or a few days should not make you feel like a failure. We all lead busy lives, and you are doing the best you can. Just look at this time as a nice pause—and when you are ready, continue doing the plan where you left off. Although this plan is meant to be implemented on thirty consecutive days, feel free to make the plan fit into your life any way you can. If it takes sixty days to do the plan and it still produces results, than that's all that matters.

6. **E-mail me.** I am here to support you. I am here to serve you. I wrote this book to help others, and I am here to help you create a better life. If you are hitting a roadblock, e-mail me and say, "Jon, I need a boost. Help me." I'll e-mail you back. People are always surprised that I return their calls and e-mails, but to me it's part of my mission and purpose. I remember e-mailing au-

thors and speakers who never contacted me back. I was crushed. I vowed I would be different. So don't be shy. I am here. E-mail me at jon@jongordon.com

Now let's get started!

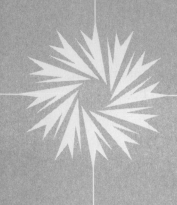

Chapter 5

The 10-Minute-a-Day Plan— Week 1

Add 10 Minutes of Positive Action to Your Day

In the last chapter, we learned just how the plan works. Now, we're ready to put it into practice. Each week, the 10-minute exercises will focus on a specific theme. This first week, we'll add 10 minutes of positive action to each day.

Because we have free will, we can take action to change our lives. Instead of struggling through life, we can flow through it. Instead of retreating from life, we can get addicted to it in a positive way. Instead of dreading tomorrow, we can look forward to enjoying each day. We don't have to move to a farm in Montana in order to reduce our stress. We don't have to wait until our vacation to be our true, happy selves. We don't have to wait until we sit on a white sandy beach to finally relax. It can start right here, right now. Life will not change without your participation, and it's certainly not going to improve unless you decide to improve it. Life doesn't change from the outside in. Our outer world merely reflects our inner world. Life changes from the inside out. So you see, change starts with us. As Gandhi suggested, we must become the change we wish to see in the world.

Habitual intention followed by habitual action creates our lives—one thought, one word, one moment, one choice, one action at a time. Each day this week you are going to habitually intend to do something. You are going to think about it and you are going to plan it. Then you are going to habitually take action. Like brushing your teeth, these habitual intentions and actions are going to become a part of your everyday life, and eventually you'll wonder how you ever lived without them. It takes only 10 minutes a day to make great things happen.

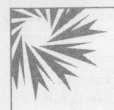

Start Your Day with a Thank-You Walk

"Happiness is produced not so much by great pieces of good fortune that seldom happen as by the little advantages that occur every day."

—Benjamin Franklin

It's simple. It's powerful. And it's a great way to kick off your thirty days of increased energy, happiness, and abundance. If in the past you have found walking to be boring, now you'll have a new way to make it fun, fresh, and meaningful. With the thank-you walk you'll be practicing the art of what I call "energy combining"—engaging in two habits that increase your energy, health, and happiness at the same time. Instead of sitting, you'll be moving. Instead of thinking about what you don't like and don't have, you'll be thinking about the gifts in your life. You'll be thinking about all the things to be grateful for. Instead of feeling stressed, you'll be feeling thankful.

When you are thankful, it's physiologically impossible to be stressed. By being thankful, you turn off your fear response system. You stop fear and stress from hijacking your mind and body, and you take control of your happiness and health. A number of studies show that grateful people tend to be more optimistic, which increases immune function and improves heart health and happiness according to Robert Emmons, a gratitude expert and professor of psychology at the University of California-Davis. Emmons's research found that people who maintained a weekly gratitude journal were more optimistic about their future, exercised more regularly, and had a greater sense of life satisfaction. In a nutshell, being thankful is good medicine and good for a happy life.

Then, when you combine walking with your thank-you's, you exponentially increase the benefits of gratitude. Walking is a powerful mental and physical energizer. When you walk, you produce endorphins and flood your brain with happy neurotransmitters such as serotonin and dopamine, which make you feel happier and more energized. So the thank-you walk helps you decrease the stress that zaps your energy and causes the release of hormones, neurotransmitters, and positive emotions that boost your energy.

SCHEDULE YOUR 10 MINUTES: Decide what time today you will do your 10-minute thank-you walk. Schedule your time now. Add it to your calendar or PDA.

Action Steps

➤ Write in your journal what you are thankful for: family, kids, your garden, the fact that you have a job, health, that you can walk, hear, etc.

➤ Find a safe place to walk.

➤ Before you walk, stretch and clear your mind.

➤ Simply start walking and say what you are thankful for. For example, I say, "I'm thankful that I am able to walk. I'm thankful that I am healthy. I'm thankful that I have a wife and children who love me. I'm thankful that I live near the beach."

➤ While you're walking, as various thoughts (besides your thankful thoughts) pop into your head, don't fight them. Just notice your thoughts and let them flow in and flow out.

➤ Refocus on being thankful. Feel thankful and this feeling will lighten your step and elevate your mood.

➤ When you are done walking, stretch. Make a mental note of how you feel.

➤ Write in your journal how you feel after your thank-you walk. (I encourage you to write down how you feel after each day's exercise, and your journal is a great place to do this.)

Note: If you are unable to walk for any reason, then simply say your thank yous while riding a stationary bike, practicing yoga, stretching, walking in a pool, or sitting in a chair. Of course, consult your doctor before beginning any exercise routine.

11th-Minute Miracle

I pray for a miracle—not any specific miracle, just a miracle that is meant to appear in my life. I pray that this plan will help me become a conduit for the miracles that are all around me. Flow through me, God, with all your miracles, love, abundance, joy, and happiness. Make me an instrument of your peace and love. Guide me to see the simple but amazing treasures hidden within me. Help me to express these gifts and receive the blessings that are meant for me. I am a miracle, and I thank you for creating me and all the miracles around me. I am ready to discover the best within me. I am ready to experience the miracles all around me. I am ready to connect with you, my higher power. I pray for a miracle. I am ready when the time is right.

Energy Foundation Tracker

I ate breakfast.	■
I ate smaller healthy meals and energizing snacks.	■
I drank plenty of water.	■
I slept enough to feel energized and rested.	■
I engaged in some form of physical activity.	■
I listened to energizing music.	■
I connected with people who increase my energy.	■
I practiced my energizer breath when stressed.	■

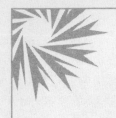

Change One Habit Today

"First we form habits, then they form us!"
—Rob Gilbert

When we think about getting healthier and more energetic, it's easy to get overwhelmed. "Where do I start?" you might ask. "How do I begin?" Well, the good news is that small changes really do yield big results. Don't think of changing your whole life overnight. Instead, just think about changing one habit. Today, you're going to make one substitution in your life—just changing one habit for one day. If you like how it feels, give it a try tomorrow, too.

I share radio tips on various radio stations around the country, called "The Energy Minute." You can hear some of these radio tips by visiting me at www.jongordon.com. The purpose of "The Energy Minute" is to provide people with simple action steps and information that will help them make small changes that produce big results. Each Energy Minute guides the listener toward action by detailing specific habits that are guaranteed to increase anyone's energy.

You'll find ten different Energy Minutes below—ten different ideas for which habit to change today. My goal for you is that you will choose just one habit to change. (If you want to change more than one habit today, that's fine, but make one habit your priority.) By just changing one small habit, you will experience the benefits and realize it is possible to change your life one energizing minute at a time. Here are ten Energy Minutes you can choose from:

1. **Replace a cup of coffee with green tea.** In addition to the health benefits of green tea (it contains antioxidants that fight cancer and help prevent heart disease), I also recommend it because it is a great alternative to coffee and caffeinated energy drinks. Green tea contains anywhere from 20 to 40 mg of caffeine, or about a quarter of the amount of caffeine in coffee. Like coffee, it gives you that energy to kick-start your day or wake you up in the afternoon. Yet green tea doesn't stimulate your body as much as coffee or other caffeinated beverages. Instead, the effects of green tea feel more like an energy boost than an energy jolt. If caffeine adversely affects you, then drink decaffeinated green tea. Just buy an organic brand that is naturally decaffeinated, using water instead of chemicals.

2. **Replace soda with water.** This one tip will increase your energy dramatically. As I wrote earlier, water is the fuel your body needs to stay energized and hydrated.

3. **Read a book instead of watching television.** While most television is passive and draining, books are alive with the energy of words—and they will fuel your life more than you could ever have imagined.

4. **Switch your candy bowl with a fruit bowl.** When you're hungry, you'll grab for whatever is available. Make it easy to make a good choice. Fruit is nature's candy, and it contains the natural sugar we crave.

5. **Take the stairs instead of the elevator at work.** Just by choosing more opportunities to walk instead of stand or sit, you will increase your metabolism and energy.

6. **Replace chips or candy bars with nuts and raisins.** Instead of processed foods, eat energizing whole-food snacks that sustain your energy.

7. **Replace your alarm clock with a rooster.** I thought of this after reading a story about a woman in New York City who had a rooster that woke up all her neighbors every morning. Okay, while you may not be able to get a rooster, do sleep with the blinds open so the sun will wake you up in the morning. Let the light be your rooster. If you are doing this plan during a time of year when there is no light in the morning, then do wake up with an alarm clock, but *don't* hit the snooze button for the next half hour. Instead, turn on all the lights and immediately get out of bed. Bright light wakes you up.

8. **Clean up your desk or car instead of leaving it cluttered.** You'll be amazed at how this makes you feel. This will clear out the stagnant energy and create more energy flow in your life.

9. **Listen instead of talking.** Instead of expending a lot of energy trying to get your point across, ask a lot of questions and let others talk while you listen. You'll find that by talking less and listening more you'll feel more energized. Plus, people will love being around you.

10. **Straighten up instead of slouching forward.** By simply straightening up and improving your posture, you change your emotional state and feel more energized. In addition, you increase your oxygen intake by up to 30 percent.

Action Steps

➤ Choose one habit from the list above and make one change today. It's that easy. Whichever habit speaks most to you is the one you should decide to change.

➤ Write down in your journal the habit you are going to change today.

➤ Focus your energy and attention on this habit.

➤ At the end of the day write down in your journal how you feel.

11th-Minute Miracle

God, grant me the strength and commitment to make positive changes in my life. For I can do great things in your strength, and I can do small acts that produce great results. Today I realize that no action is too small or insignificant. Every step leaves a footprint, and every action produces a result. Today I commit to forming good habits, and over time I will allow these habits to create my life.

Energy Foundation Tracker

I ate breakfast.	■
I ate smaller healthy meals and energizing snacks.	■
I drank plenty of water.	■
I slept enough to feel energized and rested.	■
I engaged in some form of physical activity.	■
I listened to energizing music.	■
I connected with people who increase my energy.	■
I practiced my energizer breath when stressed.	■

Week 1 Day 3

Add 3 Power Moves to Your Morning

When we build more physical muscle, it improves how we feel, think, and act. Building physical muscle is an essential component to creating a healthy and energetic *you*. Consider that every pound of muscle burns about fifty calories a day, while each pound of fat burns approximately two to three calories a day.

Weight training also revs up your metabolism in the short run as well. According to a 2001 study published in *Medicine & Science in Sports & Exercise,* when women lift weights, their metabolism remains revved up for up to two hours after the workout, burning as many as one hundred extra calories. So when you do the following three simple exercises to build more physical muscle, you'll become a calorie-burning machine after the workout and throughout the day—even while you are not exercising. And this helps you lose weight, increase your energy, and improve your health. The best part about this workout is that it takes only 10 minutes or less. These muscle-building exercises do not require weights, so you can do them anytime, anywhere.

While you are practicing these exercises, repeat the following mantra: "Every day in every way, I am feeling stronger and better." You can say this mantra out loud or silently in your mind.

How to Do It

Do one set of each exercise until muscle fatigue. You should be able to do five to thirty chair squats. Just keep doing the exercise until you feel as if your muscles have had enough.

Chair Squats *(Legs, Hamstrings, and Quads)*

With a chair behind you, stand with your feet positioned shoulder-width apart (1). Keeping your back straight and your chin up, squat down and push your rear out, as if you were sitting into the chair behind you (2). As your rear touches the chair, return to your starting position. Make sure you don't lean too far forward, which will put too much stress on your knees. Your thighs should be parallel with the floor. You should feel this exercise in your thighs, rear end, and hamstrings. You will probably be able to do five to thirty reps of this exercise. This is one of the best exercises you can do to shape up your legs and rear. To have more fun while you are doing this exercise, say, "Derriere, touch the chair."

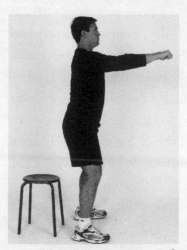

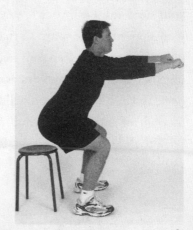

1.   2.

Push-ups
(Chest, Back, Arms)

Lie on your stomach and extend your arms and legs. Place your hands on the floor directly beneath your shoulders with your fingers facing forward (3). Balance your body on your hands and the balls of your feet. Then bend your elbows, slowly lowering your body until your chest almost touches the floor (4). Then slowly lift yourself up. **Hint:** If you are unable to do push-ups like this, use your knees to support you while you do this exercise. Or do push-ups against the wall. Don't be intimidated by push-ups. Just start small and simple and gradually build your muscles.

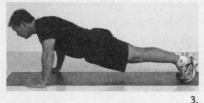
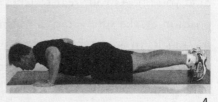

3.   4.

Abdominal Crunches

These are key for a toned tummy and powerful energy. Lie with your back on the floor and your knees bent (5). Place your hands behind your head (6). Push your lower back into the ground and slowly curl your upper body forward so that your shoulders come off the ground only a few inches. Keep your neck straight and make sure you are flexing your abdominal muscles as you crunch. The more you move your neck and head, the less you will be using your abs. Squeeze your abs for a count of one one thousand and then slowly lower your shoulders back to their starting position. Repeat until you feel a burn in your abs.

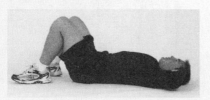
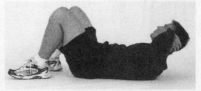

5.   6.

Jon's Energy Rule

Remember to consult with your doctor before beginning any exercise routine. If you are unable to do these exercises for any reason, then simply do the thank-you walk instead of these exercises today.

11th-Minute Miracle

God, help me choose positive energy instead of negative energy. Help me choose love instead of hate. Success instead of failure. I pray to let go of my negative thoughts, negative self-image, and self-doubt. I pray for the confidence to believe that I am a success. I pray for the strength and the patience to create a successful life, one day at a time.

Energy Foundation Tracker

I ate breakfast.	■
I ate smaller healthy meals and energizing snacks.	■
I drank plenty of water.	■
I slept enough to feel energized and rested.	■
I engaged in some form of physical activity.	■
I listened to energizing music.	■
I connected with people who increase my energy.	■
I practiced my energizer breath when stressed.	■

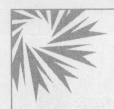

Week 1 Day 4

Breathe and Flow

One of the best ways to reclaim your energy and power is to breathe. The following exercise is designed to help you cultivate powerful, calm energy that reenergizes and recharges you. Instead of your giving away energy, this exercise will teach you how to acquire it. Instead of your scattering energy, this exercise will show you how to focus it. And instead of letting energy become stagnant in your body, this exercise will help energy move and flow through you.

This 10-minute exercise is a combination of energy breathing, qigong movements, and yoga stretches. As someone who is very busy and travels a lot, I don't have a lot of time for yoga or qigong classes; therefore I decided to combine my favorite elements from each one of these practices and create my own 10-minute exercise, which I can do anytime anywhere on a daily basis. These exercises have helped me to center and recharge my energy, and I believe they will improve your energy as well. Best of all, this routine is easy to do and it will supercharge you.

How to Do It

Energy Breathing

First, stand up straight with your hands at your sides (7). Inhale for three to four seconds as you raise your arms slowly over your head with your palms open. Your arm motion should go from your hips all the way to an outstretched position, as if you were going to give someone a big hug (8), and then over your head with your fingertips touching each other (9). Then exhale for three to four seconds as you

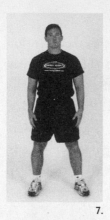
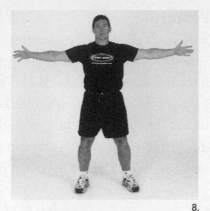
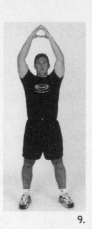

7.   8.   9.

bring your arms down, following the same motion. Repeat this for a few minutes as you focus on your breath and your body. Imagine yourself breathing in energy and calm with each inhalation and releasing stress with each exhalation.

Next, stand up straight and position your arms and your hands as if you were holding a big grapefruit in front of your belly button (10). Then exhale as you push your arms straight out in front of you, as if you were handing the big grapefruit to someone (11). Inhale as you bring the grapefruit back to the starting position in front of your belly button. Repeat this again. Exhale as you move the grapefruit away from your body and inhale as you move it toward your body.

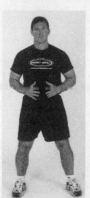
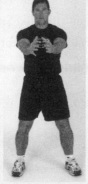

While you are exhaling and inhaling, imagine that the grapefruit you are holding is a ball of energy. Focus on this ball of energy with each breath. Do this exercise for a few moments and you will feel your energy accumulate.

Now return your arms to your side and begin a series of stretches taught to me by my yoga teacher, Nadine Bridges.

10.   11.

Mountain Posture

This pose is the basis of good posture. Starting with the attention on your feet, balance the weight of the body evenly on both sides. Pay close attention to the pressure on all four corners of the soles of the feet. Your knees should be touching, arms relaxed by your sides. Your tailbone should be lightly tucked in and your shoulders rounded backward with your shoulder blades flat against your back. Your gaze is straight ahead. Hold this for a count of four to six deep breaths.

Forward Bend

On your last deep inhale in mountain pose, raise your arms up toward the sky, reaching as high as you can (12). As you exhale, hanging from the hips and careful to keep your back as straight as possible, bend forward bringing your up-

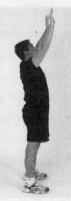 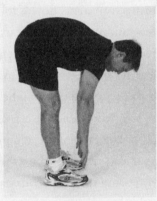

12.   13.

per torso toward your thighs (13). Don't be concerned about touching the floor, but do rest your hands where they reach comfortably. Do not bounce. Allow your body to become relaxed and heavy and hold for a count of four to six deep breaths. Slowly roll up, relaxing your knees and allowing the vertebrae to stack one on top of the other, returning to a standing position.

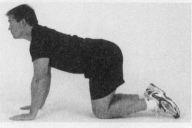 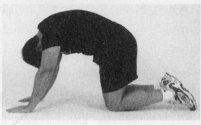

14.   15.

Table Pose/Cat and Cow Tilt

Gently make your way to the floor, coming to your hands and knees. You may want to double your mat if this hurts your knees. Your knees should be directly under your hips and hip-width apart. Your hands should be directly under your shoulders and shoulder-width apart (14). Be sure your spine is in a straight line and your head is in line with your spine. Take a few deep breaths. As you exhale, round your back up toward the sky (as your would see an angry cat do), pushing firmly down on your hands and spreading your shoulder blades wide apart. Tuck your tailbone under and draw your belly toward your spine. Allow your head to hang down, pressing your chin toward your throat. Next, as you inhale, lift your tailbone and head and create a dip in the lower back (15). Be careful not to collapse into the shoulders and keep your arms as straight as possible. Send your breath into the belly, allowing it to expand toward the floor. Turn your face up toward the sky, but keep the back of your neck soft. Move with your breath so that as you exhale you are rounding up and as you inhale you are releasing down. This is a wonderful exercise for the lower back and for focused breathing. Move between the two poses five times.

Downward Facing Dog Pose

From the Table Pose position, tuck your toes under as you exhale, lift your hips so that your body forms an upside-down V. Your hands should be flat on the floor and shoulder blades flat against your back.

Pressing firmly against the hands, bring your chest toward your thighs as you lift your tailbone toward the sky and stretch your thighs toward your hips (16). Try to keep your heels on the floor and don't worry if you need to keep your knees slightly bent. Most important is keeping the back in a nice straight

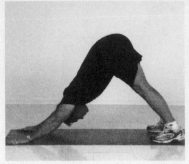

16.

line with the shoulder blades flat. Allow your head to hang and your neck to relax. Hold, using full breaths, for approximately fifteen to twenty seconds. This posture boosts circulation and is excellent for fatigue.

Child's Pose

As you exhale, slowly lower your knees to the ground returning to a tabletop position. Gently pushing against your hands lower your hips (your "sitting bones") to your heels, allowing your abdomen and chest to rest on your thighs. You may choose to keep your arms outstretched above your head or place them next to your sides with your palms facing up and relaxing your shoulders down toward the ground. Allow your forehead to rest on the

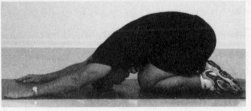

17.

ground as well (17). This pose will allow you the opportunity to explore your breath. As you inhale, feel the pressure of your belly against your thighs; you are actually massaging your internal organs. Take this opportunity to feel the breath in your back as it broadens and softens outward. Focus on the forehead against the ground, and allow your thoughts to become still. Hold this pose for as long as you feel comfortable.

Then return to a standing position and finish with a minute of energy breathing.

Note: If you are unable to do the yoga stretches for health reasons, then simply practice the energy breathing exercise for 10 minutes.

Action Steps

➤ When you are finished, write down in your journal how you feel.

11th-Minute Miracle

Dear God, with each breath I take and each move I make, I feel more connected to you, my spiritual source. So please flow through me. Allow me to feel your divine, calm energy. Help me to feel what I already know—that I am connected with all the energy and abundance around me, that I am one with everyone and everything, and that I am one with you, God. I am calm in your presence. I am centered in your peace. I am energized in your flow. Flow through me, God. I am one with you.

Energy Foundation Tracker

I ate breakfast.	▦
I ate smaller healthy meals and energizing snacks.	▦
I drank plenty of water.	▦
I slept enough to feel energized and rested.	▦

I engaged in some form of physical activity.

I listened to energizing music.

I connected with people who increase my energy.

I practiced my energizer breath when stressed.

Week 1 Day 5

Smile and Laugh

"Sometimes your joy is the source of your smile, but sometimes your smile can be the source of your joy."

—Thich Nhat Hanh

Happiness is a smile and a laugh away. University of California-San Francisco professor Paul Ekman's pioneering research on emotions revealed the universal nature of the expression of emotions. In other words, all humans share and express the same emotions . . . and these emotions create certain facial expressions. Emotions produce a certain facial expression no matter where you live or what language you speak—whether you live in a hut in New Guinea or a mansion in the United States.

According to Daniel Goleman, author of *Destructive Emotions,* Paul Ekman showed that expressions on the face offered a direct window into a person's emotions. However, Ekman's research also shows that the face not only reveals emotions but can also create them. According to Ekman, "If you intentionally make a facial expression you change your physiology. By making the correct expression you begin to have the changes in your physiology that accompany the emotion."

Thus, if we want to feel happier, we can create the facial expression that we reveal when we are happy—a smile. According to Goleman, "Simply putting the face into a smile drives the brain to activity typical of happiness—just as a frown does with sadness." In a study from Clark University in Massachusetts, when students made frowning expressions, they felt angry even when they were watching cartoons, but those who made themselves smile felt happier and enjoyed the cartoons more. So to create more happiness we need to create more smiles. We don't have to wait for something to make us smile and laugh. We can make ourselves smile whether by a funny joke, a happy memory, or a humorous story.

Norman Cousins did this and his story has become legendary. In his book *Anatomy of an Illness,* Cousins wrote about how in the 1960s he was diagnosed with a painful illness for which there was no cure. Instead of accepting his fate, he became the subject in his own experiment. He decided to fill his body with tons of positive emotions: He watched hours of Marx Brothers movies and had his nurse read him humorous stories. He discovered that a 10-minute hearty belly laugh could help him sleep two hours without pain, and in a short time he was off painkillers and sleeping pills. Cousins declared that he laughed himself to health, and research shows that he likely did. Laughter releases endorphins (our body's natural painkillers), reduces pain, boosts our immune system, increases blood circulation, reduces stress, and, as Cousins said, "Is a good way to jog internally without having to go outdoors." It appears then that happiness and better health really are a smile and a laugh away. When we are happy, we laugh and smile, but we can laugh and smile to increase our happiness. So come on and let's get happy and start smiling and laughing.

SCHEDULE YOUR 10 MINUTES: For this exercise you'll need to schedule four minutes in the morning, two minutes after lunch, two minutes after dinner, and two minutes before you go to bed. Schedule your times now. Add them to your calendar or PDA.

Action Steps

➤ In the morning, look in the mirror and think of a funny story, joke, or experience. Then smile and laugh for two minutes. This may feel a little weird, but so does taking any kind of medication for the first time. And since smiling is great natural medicine, it's worth getting used to it. Keep on thinking funny thoughts as you smile.

➤ Smile and laugh for two minutes on your way to work or when running errands. Think of the funniest movies you have ever seen.

➤ Smile for two minutes after lunch. If you work in an office, simply walk around your office smiling and saying hello to people. They won't think you're strange. They'll just think you are in a good mood.

➤ Smile and laugh for two minutes after dinner. Look in a mirror if this helps you, and think of a funny experience in your life. Or read a funny story or funny jokes.

➤ Smile for two minutes after you brush your teeth so you can see your clean teeth and increase your happiness at the same time. Think of the funniest thing that has ever happened to you.

➤ If you are not able to smile during the times I suggest, then smile when you can, whether it's a minute or five minutes at a time. The goal is to have you smile for a total of 10 minutes—however, if you want to smile even longer, then go for it.

➤ Write down how you feel. Did the smiling make you feel any happier?

11th-Minute Miracle

Today I choose happiness. I allow myself to feel happy. I allow myself to feel joy. I allow myself to laugh and smile. I allow myself to feel good. I surrender my pain, my stress, my fear, and my ego. I surrender them to you, God. I give them to you so that I may feel happy, joyful, and calm. I give you all that prevents me from connecting to you. I pray that you will flow through me. As I release my fear, stress, pain, and ego to you, I pray that you will flow through me with your joy, love, enthusiasm, and humor. Flow through me. I am ready to be a conduit for all the positive energy around me. I am ready for a miracle.

Energy Foundation Tracker

I ate breakfast.	▪
I ate smaller healthy meals and energizing snacks.	▪
I drank plenty of water.	▪
I slept enough to feel energized and rested.	▪
I engaged in some form of physical activity.	▪
I listened to energizing music.	▪
I connected with people who increase my energy.	▪
I practiced my energizer breath when stressed.	▪

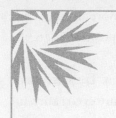

Play and Dance

"To forget oneself is to be happy."
—Robert Louis Stevenson

Now that you are feeling more energized and thankful, it's time to ignite your mind and body with the energy of play. Appropriately, while I was writing this, my four-year-old son knocked on my office door and asked if I would come play with him. As we engaged in a game of tag and catch, I both experienced and witnessed the power of play. My son was engrossed in the moment, laughing nonstop, improving his hand-eye coordination, and developing his mind and body. No wonder children seem so happy. They are always playing.

But, curiously, I also experienced these benefits within myself. I found myself concentrating on the ball, laughing when he laughed, engaged in the present moment, and having fun. I wasn't thinking about my book deadline or mortgage payment. I was playing, having fun, living life to the fullest even for a brief moment. While young animals and humans use play as a way to develop coordination, skill, and muscle, we adults can use play to train and remind our brains to have more fun and enjoy life more. The simple truth is that many of us have forgotten how to play. We allow our work, children, responsibilities, and pressures to take over our lives, and we ignore our need for fun, excitement, and laughter. We bring work home from the office, cell phones to the movies, laptops to the beach. We're working more and playing less—and this needs to change. Research shows that happy people make time for fun and enjoyment. They don't wait for it to happen, but rather they create it. Play allows us to experience a state that University of Chicago psychologist Mihaly Csikszentmihalyi termed "flow." When we are in the flow, we feel more alive, more present, and more in tune with life itself. Our stress is turned off and the flow of positive energy is turned on.

So let's stop sitting and waiting for life to happen. Let's create it. Instead of watching reality television, let's create our own reality. Instead of watching others play and have fun, let's make time for play in our own lives.

SCHEDULE YOUR 10 MINUTES. Schedule your 10 minutes of play today. Write in your journal, "I will play for 10 minutes today starting at _____ ."

Action Steps

➤ For 10 minutes, play a CD of your favorite dance music. Let go of the weight of the world and simply dance, dance, dance. If you have kids, have them dance with you. If you are by yourself, dance as wild as you would like. Or dance with your significant other. Let the energy flow and allow yourself to feel the music and let it move you.

➤ If you would like to dance for more than 10 minutes, by all means keep the energy flowing.

➤ When it's over, write down how you feel. Do you feel more alive? Do you feel happier? Write your thoughts in your journal.

11th-Minute Miracle

I am feeling more energized these days. The plan is working. So now I pray for the dedication and inspiration to keep going. God, I ask you to nudge me toward the exercises and habits I know I need to do each day to be happy. Help me stay dedicated. Help me stay focused. Help me to motivate myself. Help me discover my inner source of power that wants to shine. Help me tap this energy to make the changes I need to make and live the life I want to live. Let this energy be the spark that reignites my spirit, and let this energy be the fuel that sustains me. I am alive, God. I am energized. I am ready for continued miracles in my life.

Energy Foundation Tracker

I ate breakfast.	■
I ate smaller healthy meals and energizing snacks.	■
I drank plenty of water.	■
I slept enough to feel energized and rested.	■
I engaged in some form of physical activity.	■
I listened to energizing music.	■
I connected with people who increase my energy.	■
I practiced my energizer breath when stressed.	■

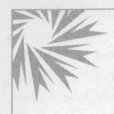

Week 1 Day 7

End your Day with a Success Walk

> "Always bear in mind that your own resolution to succeed is more important than any other one thing."
>
> —Abraham Lincoln

I found the key to life and positive energy on a golf course. Golf course, you might wonder? How could a game that makes grown men cry like babies and throw their clubs like toddlers hold the key to anything but frustration and pain? It's simple really. The amazing thing about golf, as all golfers know, is that after a round of golf you don't even remember the multitude of horrible shots you had that day. All you remember is the one great swing that landed two feet from the hole, and this memory makes you come back again and again. That's why golf is so addicting.

I couldn't help but compare this to how many of us approach life . . . but instead of focusing on the one good thing that happened to us each day, we think about the one hundred things that went wrong. Instead of thinking about our successes each day, we play our failures over and over again in our mind like a scary movie. No wonder so many of us retreat from life instead of getting addicted to it.

The key to life and positive energy, then, is to apply the one great shot golf phenomenon to your everyday life. You must remember the one great conversation, the one energizing meeting, the one act of kindness, the one great accomplishment, or the one special moment that made you smile, laugh, or cheer. No matter how difficult our days may be, I know we all have these "great moments." The key is to focus on them, remember them, and get addicted to them. Let them inspire you to wake up and take on each day just as you would a golf course. You'll go through life learning from your mistakes but remembering and focusing on your successes. Each day you'll challenge yourself to improve, grow, and have more fun. Sure, there will be days that make you want to give up, but the memory of your successes and positive experiences will motivate you to come back again and again. You'll forget the one hundred things that went wrong, and you'll remember the one thing that went right. You get addicted to the moments that make life the greatest game in the universe. You'll get addicted to life and intoxicate yourself with joy, success, positive energy, and happiness. So, to acquire this positive energy addiction, practice the success walk.

A simple 10-minute walk taken within thirty minutes of eating dinner will increase your metabolism, help you burn more calories, provide you with more nighttime energy, and help improve your sleep. So instead of plopping on the couch after dinner and falling into a food coma, take a light, easygoing walk, either by yourself or with your loved ones, and energize your evening. By focusing on your successes each day, you'll increase your optimism, and you'll create more success and positive energy in your life.

SCHEDULE YOUR 10 MINUTES sometime in the evening: Decide when you will do your 10-minute success walk this evening. Schedule your time now. Add it to your calendar or PDA.

Action Steps

➤ After dinner, spend 10 minutes walking and reflecting on your accomplishments and successes for the day. To help you focus on your accomplishments each day, complete the following sentences.

Today I consider myself a success because I _____.

Today I am proud that _____.

I had great conversations with _____.

One great thing about today was_____.

➤ This is also a great exercise to do with your children. Have them talk about their successes and accomplishments each night and you'll raise more confident children.

➤ After this exercise write down in your journal how you feel.

11th-Minute Miracle

God, I commit that I will no longer define my life by my failures. No longer will I define myself by what went wrong. I will not live in the past anymore. Today I commit to focusing on the great things that happen to me every day. While I know that success is relative, I will define my success by the great conversations I have, the wonderful people I meet, the great moments I share, and the difference I make in someone's life. Thank you for the gift of life, God. I will attempt to discover the present in each day. I am a success, God.

Energy Foundation Tracker

I ate breakfast.	■
I ate smaller healthy meals and energizing snacks.	■

I drank plenty of water.

I slept enough to feel energized and rested.

I engaged in some form of physical activity.

I listened to energizing music.

I connected with people who increase my energy.

I practiced my energizer breath when stressed.

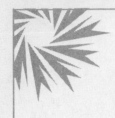

Week 1

Evaluation— Where Are You Now?

You're done with the first week of the plan. So how was it? Do you feel more alive, more focused, more positive? Complete the following scales, and let me know how you are doing. I would love to hear from you. E-mail me at jon@jongordon.com.

Negative Energy–Positive Energy Scale

| 1 | 2 | 3 | 4 | 5 | 6 | 7 | 8 | 9 | 10 |

Negative   Positive

Sad-Happy Scale

| 1 | 2 | 3 | 4 | 5 | 6 | 7 | 8 | 9 | 10 |

Sad   Happy

Stressed Scale

| 1 | 2 | 3 | 4 | 5 | 6 | 7 | 8 | 9 | 10 |

Stressed   Relaxed

Focused Scale

| 1 | 2 | 3 | 4 | 5 | 6 | 7 | 8 | 9 | 10 |

Scattered   Focused

Fear-Trust Scale

1	2	3	4	5	6	7	8	9	1 0

Fear   Trust

Overall Energy Scale

1	2	3	4	5	6	7	8	9	1 0

Low   High

Remember to visit www.jongordon.com for audio messages to inspire you as you continue with this plan.

The 10-Minute-a-Day Plan— Week 2

Add 10 Minutes of Positive Energy to Your Day

If you watch the movie *What the Bleep Do We Know?!*, which is now available on DVD, you will understand the incredible importance of your perception and how perception creates your reality. How we view the world determines the world that we see. What we think, we create. So with this book in your hands, I would like you to develop the perception that you have the power to change your life. I would like you to believe that there is happiness, joy, and positive energy inside you waiting to be discovered again and expressed. I would like you to create the belief system that your life can be happier and filled with more positive energy . . . because it can. You are about to find out that 10 minutes of positive energy and happiness can change your life.

But I'm already happy for at *least* 10 minutes each day, you may be thinking . . . and I hope that you are! But this is different. For 10 minutes each day for the next seven days, I want you to focus on being totally happy during these exercises. I want you to notice your happiness. I want you to notice how it feels and how the way you feel during those 10 minutes brings more energy and vigor into the rest of your day.

As we discussed earlier in the book, happiness really can be taught, practiced, and learned. Research demonstrates we can mold our brain to be more positive. The 10-minute-a-day exercises you are about to complete will help you choose your state of mind and your happiness. Happiness is a choice, and you are going to learn how to choose it. Instead of feeling as if you don't have a choice in life, each day you will get to choose your state of mind. You will be empowered to cultivate a state of gratitude, shift your mind-set, and change your perspective. You'll discover the power of positive emotions. You'll realize the power of connecting with others. You'll know what it feels like to feed the positive dog inside you. Instead of fretting over what you don't have, you'll learn to appreciate the gifts in your life. Instead of comparing yourself to people who are more fortunate than you, you will start to see how much you have compared to those who are less fortunate. No longer will you allow yourself to be imprisoned by your responsibilities, job, stress, fear, and past. No longer will you allow yourself to become imprisoned by what renowned psychologist Martin Seligman calls learned helplessness—a vicious cycle of mental and physical depression, fatigue, and anxiety. Dan Baker, author of *What Happy People Know* and founder of Canyon Ranch, describes Seligman's experiment:

> Seligman placed dogs individually in sealed boxes so they couldn't escape. He placed other dogs in open boxes that did allow them to escape. Then both sets of dogs were subjected to mild electrical shocks from the floor of the boxes. The dogs in the open boxes quickly learned that they could jump out to avoid the shock and did so. The dogs that were in the sealed boxes who couldn't escape soon gave up trying to get away from the shocks and just lay there, passively accepting their fates.

Seligman found that the dogs in the sealed boxes had learned to be helpless. The same dogs were then, one by one, placed in two-compartment boxes with one side safe from the shock. The dogs that were placed previously in the open boxes quickly learned to escape by going to the safe side away from the shock. However, a majority of the dogs that were previously in the sealed boxes and who had learned to feel helpless passively stayed on the side of the box that shocked them, whining with misery but passively accepting their fate. Learned helplessness in one situation had transferred to another.

Research shows that certain experiences lead to a negative thought pattern, which triggers a biochemical event in the body and the release of stress hormones. This affects energy levels, suppresses the immune system, and depletes the neurotransmitters dopamine and serotonin that make you feel happy. The result: the vicious cycle of hopelessness, anxiety, fear, and fatigue that affects millions today.

The 10-Minute-a-Day exercises this week represent the opening in the box that the dogs jumped through. You don't have to let life trap you in while you get shocked by life's struggles and challenges. You can open the box by practicing this plan and jump out when you need to. This plan demonstrates to you that you have a choice, and you can define your life rather than letting your life define you. You will create happiness 10 minutes at a time and these 10 minutes will spread happiness throughout your day and your life.

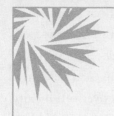

Pick a New Measuring Stick

"I cried because I had no shoes,
until I met a man who had no feet."

—Persian Proverb

"Shift your perspective," suggests Howard Cutler, coauthor of *The Art of Happiness,* a book he wrote with the Dalai Lama. According to Cutler, "We often determine our happiness by measuring ourselves against other people. We can measure ourselves against people who have more than us and say, 'We want more,' and never be happy, or we can measure it against people who have less and be thankful."

In a study performed at the State University of New York-Buffalo, one group of participants were asked to complete the sentence "I'm glad I'm not a _____," while a second group was asked by the researchers to finish the sentence "I wish I were a _____." Both groups completed the sentence five times. The group that completed the sentence "I'm glad I'm not a _____" experienced a distinct increase in life satisfaction and felt generally happier, while the second group felt more unhappy and dissatisfied with their lives. Thus a key factor in determining happiness depends on what you are using to measure your life and whom you are measuring it against. Comparing your life to the "perfect" Jones family will create jealousy, while comparing yourself to the unfortunate Smith family creates a sense of contentment.

So let's now create a new way to measure your life. Instead of thinking about what we wish we had, let's think about what we *do* have. Instead of thinking about what we don't have but want, let's think about what we are glad that we *don't* have. The 10 minutes of happiness you are about to achieve will help you choose a new measuring stick. As you shift your mind-set and perspective, you'll cultivate a greater satisfaction with your life and feel happier. And like a golfer who hits a few hundred balls a day, the more you practice these exercises the better you will get.

SCHEDULE YOUR 10 MINUTES: Decide what time today you will do your 10 minutes of happiness. Morning? Afternoon? After dinner? Schedule your time now. Add it to your calendar or PDA.

Action Steps

➤ Complete the following sentences.

I am glad that I am not a _____.

I am glad that I am not a _____.

I am glad that I am not a _____.

I am glad that I am not a _____.

I am glad that I am not a _____.

I am glad that I am not _____.

I am glad that I am not _____.

I am glad that I am not _____.

I am glad that I am not _____.

I am glad that I am not _____.

I am glad that I don't _____.

I am glad that I don't _____.

I am glad that I don't _____.

I am glad that I don't _____.

I am glad that I don't _____.

I am glad that I don't have _____.

I am glad that I don't have _____.

I am glad that I don't have _____.

I am glad that I don't have _____.

I am glad that I don't have _____.

➤ After completing all the sentences, say each sentence out loud five times.

➤ Write down in your journal how you feel now.

11th-Minute Miracle

Thank you for the gifts in my life, God. Thank you for all that I have. While my life may not be perfect and I may experience pain, I know that when I connect to you, my fear dissipates and my pain dissolves. So I connect with you now, and I thank you for all the special relationships in my life. I thank you for the ceiling over my head. I thank you for the bed that allows me to sleep and dream. I thank you for food in my refrigerator, and I thank you for the refrigerator itself. I thank you for my imperfect perfect life. I pray that my life will improve, but I accept the challenges and struggles I have been given.

I know that I am where I am right now for a reason. I am here to learn and grow, and I accept the lessons that will make me a better, stronger, happier person. Every problem brings me closer to you, God. Every challenge helps me realize I can't do it alone. So I ask for the strength to improve each day. I ask for the guidance to show me the way. Thank you for all the miracles in my life.

Energy Foundation Tracker

I ate breakfast.	◼
I ate smaller healthy meals and energizing snacks.	◼
I drank plenty of water.	◼
I slept enough to feel energized and rested.	◼
I engaged in some form of physical activity.	◼
I listened to energizing music.	◼
I connected with people who increase my energy.	◼
I practiced my energizer breath when stressed.	◼

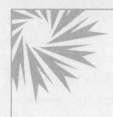

Take a Positive Energy Walk

"Our mental and emotional diets determine our overall energy levels, health, and well-being more than we realize. Every thought and feeling, no matter how big or small, impacts our inner energy reserves."

—Doc Childre

The 10-minute positive energy walk is a powerful combination of physical activity that increases your endorphins, blood flow, and energy. Emotions are powerful charges of energy that can lift us up or take us down a spiral staircase of sadness. If you have ever had one of those days when a mood just came over you like a black cloud and you felt down, depressed, or in a funk for no apparent reason, then you know how emotions can affect you. They can make you excited and euphoric or angry and violent. Emotions often control what you think, say, and do, and affect your physiology in the process.

Research shows that we can change our emotional state by changing our physiology. Just the act of standing up tall instead of being slouched over will change the way you feel and think. Try it and see for yourself. We can also positively charge our emotions through our thoughts and words. Emotional energy not only flows from emotion to action but also from action to emotion. Just as certain emotions cause us to think, say, and act a particular way, we can create emotions by thinking, saying, and acting in ways that trigger these emotions. Instead of letting our emotions control us, we can take control of our emotions—which is essential when creating happiness and positive energy.

So today let's take some action and create positive emotions through your thoughts and words. Remember, the more you take action to cultivate positive emotions, the more automatic this emotional response will become. Instead of letting negative emotions take hold of you, by practicing this exercise you will be able to take hold of your emotions and create more happiness and positive energy in your life. Together, the act of walking combined with the following positive energy boosters creates one of my favorite exercises, and it is something I do on a daily basis.

SCHEDULE YOUR 10 MINUTES: Decide what time today you will do your 10-minute positive energy walk. Morning? Afternoon? After dinner? Schedule your time now. Add it to your calendar or PDA. **Hint:** This makes a great exercise to kick-start your day.

Action Steps

➤ Start walking. Make sure you are walking tall with your posture straight. Arch your shoulders and walk as if you are very confident. Even the way you walk affects your emotions. Slouch over and you'll feel blah. Stand straight and you feel better. So walk tall.

➤ While you are walking, start saying your emotional energy boosters.

➤ Repeat the following emotional energy booster for two minutes. "Every day in every way, I increase my energy. *Yes!* Every day in every way, I increase my energy. *Yes!*"

➤ Now repeat the following statement for two minutes. "I was born to energize. *Yes!* I was born to energize. *Yes!*" While you are saying this, realize that you were born to energize yourself, your friends, your community, your family, and your coworkers.

➤ Then, for two minutes, say the following: "Every day in every way I'm feeling stronger and happier. *Yes!* Every day in every way, I'm feeling stronger and happier. *Yes!*"

➤ For two minutes say the following: "Yes, yes, yes, I am a success. Yes, yes, yes. I am a success."

➤ Finally, for two minutes, say, "Great things are happening. Yes. Great things are happening. Yes."

➤ Although I recommend saying each sentence for two minutes, if there is one emotional energy booster you like more than others (or you don't resonate with one of the sentences and you want to leave it out), then just pick the one you like the best and say it for 10 minutes while walking. Choose the boosters that work best for you.

➤ I also encourage you to write and say your own energy boosters based on whatever it is you want to create in your life. So, for example, if one of your intentions is to create more financial abundance, you might write and say, "I am abundant, healthy, wealthy, and successful. I have all that I need right now." Simply write and say what inspires you and emotionally charges you, and let the energy flow.

➤ When you finish this exercise, write down in your journal how you feel.

Remember to consult with your doctor before beginning any exercise routine. If you are unable to walk for any reason, then simply charge up your emotions while riding a stationary bike, stretching, walking in a pool, or sitting in a chair.

11th-Minute Miracle

Dear God, allow me to see that I am whole. I am not my weaknesses, problems, or worries. I am my strengths. Help me to use these 10-minute exercises to find the best in me, and then let me embody this feeling throughout the day, week, month, and year. When I am weak, let me remember that I am strong. When I am sad, remind me why I should be happy. When I fear, let me transition to trust. When I feel the urge to hate, fill my heart with compassion. When I am negative, help me be positive. Give me strength, God. Allow me to see through new eyes that I am whole, that I am strong, that I am positive—that I am loved by you.

Energy Foundation Tracker

I ate breakfast.	■
I ate smaller healthy meals and energizing snacks.	■
I drank plenty of water.	■
I slept enough to feel energized and rested.	■
I engaged in some form of physical activity.	■
I listened to energizing music.	■
I connected with people who increase my energy.	■
I practiced my energizer breath when stressed.	■

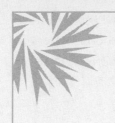

Week 2 Day 10

Feed the Positive Dog

"Some pursue happiness—others create it."
—Anonymous

Earlier in the book we discussed the story about "feeding the positive dog inside us" and starving the negative dog. Well, now it's time to apply this story to your life and feed the positive dog inside you. Instead of thinking about everything that you don't have, don't like, and don't want, it's now time to think about everything that is great in your life. It's time to list great things about yourself.

Identify your good characteristics. What are your strengths? What is the one good thing about your life? In my coaching I have found that when we are thinking about the great things, we are not thinking about the things we don't like. Two thoughts cannot occupy the same place in your mind. When we feed the positive dog, it grows and grows. Each time you think about what is great in your life, you'll be creating more optimism, a stronger immune system, and a happier you. Amazingly, every time I do these exercises in my seminars people get nervous at first. It's like they don't know what to say. Yet if I asked them what is not good in their lives, they could rattle off a twenty-minute speech. This is precisely the pattern feeding the positive dog exercise is meant to change. The great news is that as people do this exercise during my seminar, nervousness dissipates and a lighter, freer energy flows. It changes the energy of each person, and an incredible shift is felt in the room. Well, now its time to create your energy shift. It starts with the following 10 minutes.

SCHEDULE YOUR 10 MINUTES: Decide what time today you will do your 10 minutes of happiness. Morning? Afternoon? After dinner? Schedule your time now. Add it to your calendar or PDA.

Action Steps

➤ Complete the following sentences:

I am happy that I have a _____.

I am happy that I have a _____.

I am happy that _____.

I am happy that_____.

I am thankful that I am _____.

I am thankful that I am_____.

I am thankful that I have_____.

I am thankful that I have_____.

➤ Answer the following sentences:

Three great things I like about myself are

1._____

2._____

3._____

My three strengths are

1. _____

2. _____

3. _____

I can use these strengths in my life by doing:

_____

_____

Three of my most meaningful accomplishments were

1. _____

_____

2. _____

_____

3. _____

_____

➤ Read each sentence aloud.

➤ Write down how you feel after doing these exercises.

11th-Minute Miracle

I pray for abundance, God. I accept all the joy, health, happiness, love, passion, and purpose in my life. I am one with you, God, and like a river running into the ocean, I allow myself to connect to you, for you are my source. I know that when I connect to you, I become part of everyone and everything in the universe. I become one with all the energy and abundance that exists. So I pray for abundance, and I accept this abundance in my life. I am open to it, and I allow myself to receive it. Thank you for all the abundance in my life.

Energy Foundation Tracker

I ate breakfast.	■
I ate smaller healthy meals and energizing snacks.	■
I drank plenty of water.	■
I slept enough to feel energized and rested.	■
I engaged in some form of physical activity.	■
I listened to energizing music.	■
I connected with people who increase my energy.	■
I practiced my energizer breath when stressed.	■

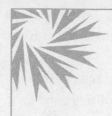

Remember Your Greatest Moment

"We are not powerless specks of dust
drifting around in the wind, blown by
random destiny. We are, each of us, like
beautiful snowflakes—unique, and born
for a specific reason and purpose."

—Elisabeth Kübler-Ross

If I asked you to describe your greatest moment, what would you say? Perhaps you would tell me about the birth of your child. Or the moment you were married. For some it might even be the day you were divorced. (I hear this often in my seminars. It sounds funny, but for many it's true!) It might be the time you saved someone's life or gave the best performance of your life. You may tell me about the time you fell in love, graduated from school, experienced a major breakthrough, or the time that all of your hard work paid off. And perhaps there are several great moments that make it impossible to pick just one.

I ask you to think about these moments because when we are dealing with a stressful or fearful event in our life (or simply a stressful day), one of the best ways to overcome this stress and fear is to fuel up with positive energy by thinking of a great memory. As I've stressed repeatedly, when our brain is focused on something positive, it's not thinking about a negative. Even more important is the fact that the more you think about something positive, the more your brain automatically thinks positively. It becomes a habit. So whatever your greatest moment is or whether you have many great moments, I encourage you to write them down. Then I encourage you to think about them whenever you are feeling a little down or stressed. Let these moments be the positive energy that helps you get up in the morning and take a walk. Let them create a smile on your face, a gleam in your eye, and a feeling of joy throughout your body. Allow these moments to help you overcome life's challenges and flow through the day. Let them inspire you to get through a difficult project or task.

Let these moments remind you of what is truly important. For it's not the number of moments we live that matters but the quality of the moments that define our life. We can't control what happens to us, but we can control what we think about. Positive energy is a choice, then, and what we choose to think about determines how we see our life and our world. We can define our life by our dramas or our successes. Those who think of their great moment and successes are simply . . . happier. So I ask you again, "What is your greatest moment?"

SCHEDULE YOUR 10 MINUTES: Decide what time today you will do your 10 minutes of positive energy. Morning? Afternoon? After dinner? Schedule your time now. Add it to your calendar or PDA.

Action Steps

➤ Think about your life and identify your top three greatest moments.

➤ Write them down in your journal. Describe them as vividly as you can.

➤ Spend a few minutes visualizing your greatest moments. Close your eyes and picture the moment happening as if it were today.

➤ After this exercise, write down in your journal how you feel.

11th-Minute Miracle

I surrender my need for approval, God. I let go of my ego that wants approval from others and wants to be important. I realize that all I have to do is shine for you, God. All I have to do is shine my light, my positive energy, my passion, my enthusiasm, and my gifts that you have given me. All I have to do is shine for you, God. It doesn't matter what others think. All I have to do is shine for you and share my gifts with the world. All I have to do is share the happiness and joy that exist within me. I've never found happiness in trying to please others. Now I know that if I find the light inside me and let it shine, then I will be happy. And I know that if I am happy, I will be successful. Others will see my light and they will want to be around it. They will want to bask in it. And when they ask me where this power and strength came from, I will gladly tell them so they too can share their gifts with the world. So instead of living from the outside in, I choose to live from the inside out, with a light that shines for you and shines on others.

Energy Foundation Tracker

I ate breakfast.	■
I ate smaller healthy meals and energizing snacks.	■
I drank plenty of water.	■
I slept enough to feel energized and rested.	■
I engaged in some form of physical activity.	■
I listened to energizing music.	■
I connected with people who increase my energy.	■
I practiced my energizer breath when stressed.	■

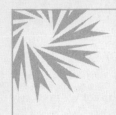

Start Your Day with Positive Words

"Everything you are against weakens you.
Everything you are for empowers you."
—Dr. Wayne Dyer

As Emerson states, "The ancestor to every action is a thought." To create a life filled with positive energy, you must create thoughts and words filled with positive energy. Energy comes before matter, and if you want to change your physical reality, you must change your energy. Thoughts and words are energy, and to change your energy, you must change your thoughts and words. Thoughts can fuel us positively or negatively. They can strengthen us or weaken us. The choice is ours. We can choose to fuel our lives with positive thoughts and words that energize us, or we can allow self-doubt and negative self-talk to tear us down.

Think of your thoughts and words as the gas that keeps your engine running. An abundant source of great fuel will take you wherever you desire. On the other hand, dirty fuel will clog your system and leave you stranded—wondering about the places you could have been. The good news is that you don't have to wonder because this exercise will provide you with the fuel to take you where you want to go. It starts where everything begins—with our thoughts and words. Let's fuel up with positive thoughts and words and positive energy. The best time to fuel up is in the morning.

SCHEDULE YOUR 10 MINUTES sometime in the morning: Decide when you will do your 10 minutes of positive energy this morning. Schedule your time now. Add it to your calendar or PDA.

Action Steps

➤ Read the following sentences to fuel up with positive thoughts and words. **Hint:** You can also do this exercise while walking.

> ➤ I am focused today. I am like a laser ready to focus on what I need to do to create success today.
>
> ➤ I am positive today. I am a powerful force of positive energy.
>
> ➤ I am happy. Today I allow myself to experience happiness.
>
> ➤ I am relaxed today. I feel calm energy and it feels great.
>
> ➤ I am optimistic today. I believe great things are happening.
>
> ➤ I accept all the great things that happen today.
>
> ➤ I accept all the great people I meet today.
>
> ➤ I accept all the great conversations I have today.
>
> ➤ I accept all the health, wealth, success, joy, and abundance in my life today.
>
> ➤ I look forward to the rest of the day.
>
> ➤ I look forward to the people I am going to meet.
>
> ➤ I look forward to the things I am going to learn.
>
> ➤ I look forward to the successes I am creating.

➤ Repeat the phrases above several times with enthusiasm and positive energy. Feel the energy of the words, and let them ignite you.

➤ Now take a few sheets of computer paper and on each sheet write in big letters:

I LOVE LIFE

➤ Post these sheets on your bathroom mirror, your car dashboard, and your desk if you work in an office. Let the phrase "I love life" remind you to fuel up with positive energy during your day.

➤ After this exercise, write down in your journal how you feel.

11th-Minute Miracle

Today I ask you, God, to make me a conduit for your miracles. Allow me to experience miracles in my life, and use me to show others the potential for miracles in their lives. Make me a conduit for your love, joy, compassion, passion, purpose, and positive energy. Make me an expression of your positive energy. Allow me to be contagious and share this positive energy with others. Help me shine on all those who come into contact with me. Use me to help people see miracles. Guide me to help others create miracles. Make me an instrument of your peace, and allow me to cocreate a more positive world with you. I am ready to serve with positive energy, God. The world needs more of it, and I am ready to create it and share it. Thank you for this gift.

Energy Foundation Tracker

I ate breakfast.	▣
I ate smaller healthy meals and energizing snacks.	▣
I drank plenty of water.	▣
I slept enough to feel energized and rested.	▣
I engaged in some form of physical activity.	▣

I listened to energizing music.

I connected with people who increase my energy.

I practiced my energizer breath when stressed.

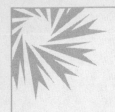

Try Something New

> "Sing like no one is listening, dance like no one is watching, love like you'll never get hurt, and live like it's heaven on earth."
>
> —Anonymous

Now it's time to engage in some new playful activity that will increase your happiness. Gregory Berns, M.D., associate professor of psychiatry and behavioral sciences at Emory University, believes that novelty is the key to a satisfying life. He believes when humans constantly try new challenges and adventures, it makes us happier. He's not necessarily talking about skydiving or climbing Mount Everest, but rather stimulating experiences that make us feel engaged or in the flow. Several activities he has people engage in include trying a new sport or fitness activity, reading a new novel, and attending a lecture on an unfamiliar subject. Based on Berns's research and on the old adage that "variety is the spice of life," my goal for you today is that you will try something new. You will engage in an activity that you have not done before. You will fuel your life with a new experience and energy, and this energy will boost your mood and increase your happiness.

SCHEDULE YOUR 10 MINUTES. Decide when you will engage in your 10 minutes of play today. Add it to your calendar or PDA.

Action Steps

➤ Because a "new" activity is considered different for each of us, I want you to pick one of the following activities and play for 10 minutes.

➤ Using three tennis balls, try to juggle. Even if it feels awkward, try to juggle for 10 minutes. Hold two balls in your left hand and one in your right hand. Throw one of the balls in your left hand up in the air. As that ball is in the air then release the ball in your right hand in the air and try to catch the first ball with your right hand. Just when you catch it with your right hand, you should release the ball in your left hand into the air and so on. For a visual of how to juggle, visit www.acm.uiuc.edu/webmonkeys/juggling. Have fun.

➤ Buy a hula hoop and try to keep it above your waist. Keep practicing for 10 minutes.

➤ Go to your favorite bookstore and search for different kinds of books that you are normally not interested in. Buy a book within 10 minutes and commit to reading it.

➤ Get a bouncy ball from a toy store and try to bounce it as many times as you can without its rolling away from you.

➤ In 10 minutes, write a short country song about your life. Make it as funny as you like.

➤ Ride a bicycle if you own one and haven't ridden it in over five years.

➤ Try a new recipe, something you have never made before.

➤ Call one of your favorite local radio stations, and ask them to play one of your favorite songs.

➤ Get some Play-Doh or Legos and create whatever comes to mind.

➤ Do something you have always wanted to do but have never tried.

11th-Minute Miracle

Dear God, I want to thank you for bringing this plan into my life. It is no accident that I came across this plan, and I look forward to incorporating many of the things I have learned. I ask you to help me stay on course. Help me to stay calm and focused—to be positive and confident—to trust in myself and my future. I want to become a better person each day, and with your support I know I can do it. I am prepared to continue to improve my life one day at a time. Thank you for your blessings. Thank you for the gifts you have given me. Thank you for my life. I am ready to shine.

Energy Foundation Tracker

I ate breakfast.	■
I ate smaller healthy meals and energizing snacks.	■
I drank plenty of water.	■
I slept enough to feel energized and rested.	■
I engaged in some form of physical activity.	■
I listened to energizing music.	■
I connected with people who increase my energy.	■
I practiced my energizer breath when stressed.	■

Get Connected with Others

"A friend is a present you give yourself."
—Robert Louis Stevenson

If you want to be happier, don't try to make more money. Instead, make more friends. According to David Myers, author of *The Pursuit of Happiness,* research demonstrates that once middle-class comforts are in place, there is a very weak link between happiness and income. And as nations grow wealthier, there is no sign of increased happiness. In fact, rates of depression and alcoholism have increased in the United States since World War II, even though we have experienced the greatest period of economic growth ever. The old adage that money doesn't buy happiness clearly rings true.

However, being rich in friends certainly does make a difference. According to a survey from the National Opinion Research Center, the more friends you have the happier you are. Other studies show that close relationships promote health, and according to Robert D. Putnam, Ph.D., author of *Better Together: Restoring the American Community,* "Your chances of dying in the next twelve months are halved by joining a group." He says, "Social isolation is as big a risk factor for death as smoking, and by far the biggest component of happiness is how connected you are." So instead of constantly chasing the dollar, you may want to consider making more time to reach out and connect with others. As is the case with every strategy in this book, we don't have to take a lot of time to see the benefits of our actions. We can make quality and meaningful connections in short periods of time. It is better to connect with someone for 10 minutes than to wait a year till you have an hour to spend with them. So enjoy the exercise for today and get connected.

SCHEDULE YOUR 10 MINUTES: Decide what time today you will do your 10 minutes of positive energy. Morning? Afternoon? After dinner? Schedule your time now. Add it to your calendar or PDA.

Action Steps

➤ Choose one of the following exercises to connect with someone who increases your positive energy.

1. Ask a friend, neighbor, or family member to take a thank-you walk with you. While you walk with your partner, have each of you state what you are thankful for while the other person listens.
2. Call up an old friend who always makes you laugh and smile.
3. Write a few meaningful cards to friends or family members who you haven't spoken to or seen in a while. Don't do this via e-mail. Rather, do it the old-fashioned way with paper, pen, and envelope. You'll be amazed at how refreshing it feels.
4. Tonight, walk outside in your neighborhood and ask your neighbors how they are doing. If you are like one of the women in my seminars who said that she lived in a crime-ridden neighborhood and couldn't do this, then simply call a few of your neighbors on the phone and ask if they are all right.

➤ Write down how you feel after you have connected with others.

11th-Minute Miracle

I pray for the confidence and the energy to reach out and connect with others. I know that when I connect I am benefiting not only the health of another person but my own health as well. I ask for the compassion to be there when others need me. I ask for the strength to take action and help them. I ask for the selflessness to put the needs of others before my own. I know that when I serve others, I am also serving you, God. I am serving a bigger purpose and tapping into an infinite amount of energy that is available to me. And when I connect, I bring this infinite energy into my life and the lives of others. Most of all, thank you for all the people you have brought and will bring into my life. I accept these wonderful connections, and I commit to creating more of them.

Energy Foundation Tracker

I ate breakfast.	▪
I ate smaller healthy meals and energizing snacks.	▪
I drank plenty of water.	▪
I slept enough to feel energized and rested.	▪
I engaged in some form of physical activity.	▪
I listened to energizing music.	▪
I connected with people who increase my energy.	▪
I practiced my energizer breath when stressed.	▪

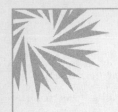

Week 2

Evaluation— Where Are You Now?

You're completed the second week of the plan. You are at the midpoint. So how was it? Do you feel more alive, more focused, more positive? Complete the following scales, and let me know how you are doing. I would love to hear from you. E-mail me at jon@ jongordon.com.

Negative Energy–Positive Energy Scale

1	2	3	4	5	6	7	8	9	10

Negative   Positive

Sad-Happy Scale

1	2	3	4	5	6	7	8	9	10

Sad   Happy

Stressed Scale

1	2	3	4	5	6	7	8	9	10

Stressed   Relaxed

Focused Scale

1	2	3	4	5	6	7	8	9	1 0

Scattered   Focused

Fear-Trust Scale

1	2	3	4	5	6	7	8	9	1 0

Fear   Trust

Overall Energy Scale

1	2	3	4	5	6	7	8	9	1 0

Low   High

Chapter 7

The 10-Minute-a-Day Plan— Week 3

Lose 10 Minutes of Negative Energy in Your Day

At this point in the plan you most likely feel happier and more energized. However, if you are like most people, there is still something holding you back. You don't feel as great as you could. You know you can feel even better, but you're not quite sure how. After all, you can't move forward if you don't know what is holding you back.

Let me introduce you to the power of letting go. As I mentioned earlier in the plan, we all have sludge (or what I call "energy blockers") that clog up our energy pipeline. These energy blockers include fear, stress, negative people, emotional pain, self-doubt, and living in the past. They are sources of negative energy that weigh us down mentally, physically, emotionally, and spiritually. They cause resistance in us and keep us from reaching our full potential.

In fact, a woman who was implementing the 10-Minute-a-Day Plan e-mailed me recently that "although I do feel more positive, I still feel like I am just sugar-coating the negativity inside me." I e-mailed her back that I couldn't agree more. I said to create a more powerful transformation in our lives, we must spend time letting go of negative energy to make room as we fill up with positive energy. They go hand in hand. When you let go and lose 10 minutes of negative energy in your day, you release the energy blockers and you allow more positive and abundant energy to flow into your life. We must let go so we can charge up.

If I didn't offer this week's exercises, this plan would not be complete. And if we don't practice letting go, our life will not be complete. The key is to let go through your thoughts, words, breath, and actions. I personally practice these exercises every day and have experienced amazing results in my life. If this concept of "letting go" is new to you, you'll soon realize that these exercises are actually very easy. Get your Liquid Drano ready. It's time to clear out your energy pipeline.

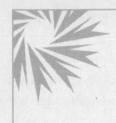

Neutralize Your Energy Terminators

As I wrote about earlier in the book, too much technology, or what I call "energy terminators," is draining our energy and causing the stress that clogs up our energy pipeline. So as you begin to let go this week, the first step I want you to take is to neutralize your energy terminators and eliminate the power they have over you. It may not be easy, but when you lose the 10 minutes of negative energy these energy terminators cause in your life, you will feel energized and free once again.

It's a challenge I know all too well. While on a multicity book and speaking tour, I realized how great I felt. I was appearing on television shows, meeting people at book signings and readings, and writing on planes. Rarely was I on my computer, and I felt great. But when I returned to a computer . . . hundreds of e-mails awaited me, and my voice mail was full. The more time I spent on my computer answering questions and responding to e-mails, the worse I felt. I started having trouble sleeping and found it impossible to slow down and relax. I became consumed with the nagging feeling that I "must" check my e-mail every few minutes, that I must answer every cell phone call regardless of whether I was spending time with family. I was doing everything that, as an energy coach, I teach people *not* to do!

It got so bad that my body finally broke down, and I became very ill. While recovering for several weeks, I had a lot of time to think, and I finally made the connection between how I felt when I was traveling (limiting technology and information) and how I felt when

I was always plugged in and connected. Like all problems, this one was a gift that has made me wiser and stronger.

Now my mission is to share what I know about how to overcome the T.I.R.E.D. Syndrome I discussed earlier and neutralize the energy terminators. While we can't change our society, we can change our habits and the way we use technology and information. These techniques worked for me, and I believe they will work wonders for you. Today, neutralize your energy terminators by taking the following action steps.

Action Steps

➤ **Use your personal "off" button.** All of our machines have them, and we need one, too. The amount of information available to us will only continue to increase as the speed of technology accelerates. Therefore it is up to each one of us to manage our power source and shut down.

For instance, on the *Today* show I coached Audrey Dorsey, a divorced mother of two, to stop checking her e-mail every night at seven. Before this, she would answer e-mails well into midnight. Once she incorporated this simple strategy, she went to bed earlier, got more sleep, and felt much more energized and relaxed in the morning. It increased her productivity tenfold. So set a stop time when you will stop using your computer today and stop answering calls. Remember, you are like a computer. If you're left on 24/7, you will eventually overheat and burn out.

➤ **Make technology work for you.**
  ➤ Shut off the cell phone when you are driving home from work today. Use that time to unwind, breathe deeply, and release tension and stress.
  ➤ Shut off your cell phone when you go to meet a friend for lunch or go to the movies or eat out in a restaurant.

➤   Ignore the call-waiting feature. Focus your energy on the person you are talking to. They'll feel better and so will you. You can check your voice mail and return your calls later. Realize that you are the boss, and your phone works for you. Shut it off whenever you want some peace and quiet.

➤   Use voice mail and caller ID. Talk when you are ready to talk. Otherwise, let the caller leave a message and respond when you are ready.

➤   **Cure your e-mail addiction.** Limit the number of times you check your e-mail today. I now check my e-mail three times a day instead of twenty, and I am much more productive, focused, and relaxed. Schedule your times. For instance, my times are noon, three, and eight. Determine your most productive times of the day and *don't* use e-mail during this time. Instead of constantly checking your e-mails and responding to the world, you'll start creating it. Schedule three times to check your e-mail today.

➤   **Get off your dot.com chair and take a walk in nature.** One of the easiest and simplest things we can do to neutralize our energy terminators is to run away and refuel with nature. While computers zap your energy, nature restores it. In fact, a recent client just received a promotion at work after making time for 10-minute walks outside during her lunch break. She was so much more productive and positive her company couldn't help but notice her change in behavior and attitude . . . and they recognized her for it.

➤   Describe how you feel at the end of the day. Write your feelings in your journal.

11th-Minute Miracle

Dear God, help me to regain power over my life. Help me to become a master of my technology-filled world. Because, as we know, real power does not come from a machine but rather by plugging into your ultimate power. While I often try to search for the answers online, God, today I commit to finding more moments of stillness and letting you provide me with the search results I seek. You are the ultimate search engine, and today I pray for your guidance and the answers I need to know at this time in my life.

Energy Foundation Tracker

I ate breakfast.	▪
I ate smaller healthy meals and energizing snacks.	▪
I drank plenty of water.	▪
I slept enough to feel energized and rested.	▪
I engaged in some form of physical activity.	▪
I listened to energizing music.	▪
I connected with people who increase my energy.	▪
I practiced my energizer breath when stressed.	▪

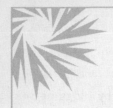

Week 3 Day 16

Lose 10 Minutes of Busyness

"When you're in solitary confinement and
you're six feet under without light, sound,
or running water, there is no place to go but
inside. And when you go inside, you discover
that everything that exists in the universe
is also within you."

—Rubin Carter, aka "The Hurricane"

For the past fifteen days you have engaged in exercises that helped you positively shift your active mind and thoughts. You have shifted from sadness to happiness, negative energy to positive energy, and craving to gratitude. Each of these exercises helped you shift your thinking and mind-set. Now I want to help you engage in an entirely different exercise that will not shift your thinking but rather help quiet your thinking and calm your mind.

In my book *Energy Addict*, I wrote the following: "My house is quiet. The kids are asleep and the world is silent, if only for a brief moment. Yet it is in these brief moments that the energy sits, waiting to be tapped, where ideas originate and out of nothing flows everything. . . . Within the silence sits the energy to recharge our batteries—to refuel our tired lives, to help us create." Today I believe in this statement more than ever. In our noisy, chaotic, busy lives, silence is the medicine we need to heal, to recharge, to reenergize.

For the last several years I have talked with many moms who have small children, as well as with CEOs who oversee thousands of employees. I've instructed all these people to simply take 10-minute breaks to allow themselves a few minutes of silence in their days. The results cannot be denied. They all feel refreshed, recharged, and refocused to take on the rest of the day—and so can you. You just have to commit to 10 minutes of silence. I warn you, though, that this is not easy. It may be one of the most difficult tasks in this plan. We have become so addicted to "doing" and "achieving" that we have forgotten how to just "be" and "rest."

At first you may feel like jumping out of your skin. If this is the case, know that you need this exercise more than anyone, and you are someone who needs to lose your busyness and become busy-less. Everything in nature requires time for renewal and growth. If you are always giving and expending energy but not taking the time to renew and recharge, then your energy system will break down. So I urge you to resist the urge to get up and say, "I just can't sit and relax." Work through the discomfort of "being" and know that it is what you need the most, and when you take time to sit in silence, you heal your heart and soul and you recharge your life battery. So today lose your busyness and bring on the silence.

SCHEDULE YOUR 10 MINUTES OF SILENT ENERGY today. What time will you take this energy break? Commit to it! Write the time of day or specific time in your journal.

Action Steps
➤ Find a quiet place. Perhaps it's your office or bedroom or a park bench outside your office. Sit in a comfortable position.

➤ Start focusing on your breathing—inhaling through your nose and exhaling through your nose and mouth. (If you have trouble breathing through your nose, breathe through your nose and mouth.) Focus on your breath as it lifts the belly and follow it as it lifts your diaphragm, chest, and then shoulders. Focus on your breath as you exhale and it leaves your body. Relax and let your breath get quieter and lighter. Continue to focus on your breathing.

➤ As you inhale and exhale, visualize your favorite place. Perhaps it's a beach, the mountains, a village in Europe, or a park in your town. Hold this picture in your mind as you focus on your breathing. See the vivid details of your favorite place as you inhale and exhale.

➤ As thoughts come into your mind, don't fight them. Let them flow in and flow out. Focus on your breathing and your favorite place. If you get distracted, just stop, relax, and return to the second step. This exercise will get easier and easier as you practice it.

➤ Continue this process for 10 minutes. You'll be amazed how fast 10 minutes pass. Understand that if you are new to this exercise, it will feel a little awkward at first, but after a little practice it will feel quite natural.

➤ After this exercise write down in your journal how you feel.

11th-Minute Miracle

Help me relax, God, so that I can sit peacefully and quietly. Help me tune out the world so I can take refuge and focus on my inner strength. Help me remember this powerful moment of silence as I go through my day. Help me use this quiet time to improve my life and the lives of those I touch today. Help me remember this peaceful feeling when a stressful event occurs. Help me be the person I know

I was born to be. Help me to be the calm I wish to see more of in the world.

Energy Foundation Tracker

I ate breakfast.	▪
I ate smaller healthy meals and energizing snacks.	▪
I drank plenty of water.	▪
I slept enough to feel energized and rested.	▪
I engaged in some form of physical activity.	▪
I listened to energizing music.	▪
I connected with people who increase my energy.	▪
I practiced my energizer breath when stressed.	▪

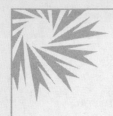

Lose an Energy Vampire

"I will not let anyone walk through my mind with their dirty feet."

—Gandhi

As we discussed earlier in the book, there are people who increase your energy and those who drain your energy. While it is important to surround yourself with positive and supportive people, we must also address how to deal with the people who bring us down. So the goal today is to lose an energy vampire and lose the negative energy you feel when you are around them. There are three ways to lose an energy vampire.

1. **Run away as fast as you can whenever you see them.** Lose them so they can't find you. If you hide for 10 minutes, they will go away. While this sounds funny, sometimes it is necessary to preserve your precious energy.

2. **Confront and reform.** The first step is to hold up a mirror. You need to find out if they even realize they are an Energy Vampire. While normal vampires can't see their reflection, energy vampires can often see the vampire within them once you show them. This is the confrontation part. Tell them they are being negative and help them change. Tell them they are an energy vampire in a loving, nonjudgmental way, and explain how they make you feel. Then reform them—encourage them to enter a positive energy addiction program. Positive energy is the only addiction worth

having. Help them become an Energy Addict by reading my book *Energy Addict: 101 Physical, Mental, and Spiritual Ways to Energize Your Life,* and have them follow this plan.

3. **Neutralize them.** Not with stakes or garlic but with kindness. In many life and work situations it's not possible to run or confront. For example, if your boss is an energy vampire, you may not want to (or be able to) say anything. These situations, while very difficult, often provide us with our most powerful lessons. They teach us that we must lose the negative energy within ourselves and cultivate more positive energy. To kill energy vampires with kindness, it doesn't mean you fake a smile when you are around them, but rather you shine on them with your love, compassion, and positive energy. You realize they are negative people who are suffering, and while they may be mean or miserable, you have compassion for them. Just as a germ gets neutralized by your immune system, your love and empathy is the cure for the common energy vampire. As Walt Whitman said, "You will convince by your presence." Most of all, you will learn that someone's negativity can affect you only if you allow it to. During week 4 of this plan you will practice several exercises that will help you stay strong and positive in the face of negativity.

Now that you know how to lose an energy vampire, the plan is to take action by using one of these strategies. Practice the following action steps today:

SCHEDULE YOUR 10 MINUTES OF ENERGY VAMPIRE NEUTRALIZING. Schedule your time now. Add it to your calendar or PDA.

Action Steps

➤ Look in the mirror: Sometimes we think others are negative, but it is we who are the energy vampires. Take a positive energy inventory of yourself. Are you doing all you can do to share positive energy? Are you being judgmental? Is there something you can do differently that would change the situation?

➤ Identify the energy vampires in your life.

➤ Decide which strategy you will use on them. Use the energy vampire neutralizing planner to help you during this process.

Energy Vampire	Neutralizing Strategy	Did it Work? Comments
1.		
2.		
3.		

➤ Take action.
➤ Write down at the end of the day how you felt. Did it work?

11th-Minute Miracle

God, I pray for the strength to overcome the forces of negativity in my life. Make me a conduit for your love and compassion. Use me to shine on others who are in pain, fear, and doubt. Help me to heal these people with my presence. Use me to create more smiles, more joy, more energy, and more happiness wherever I go and help me to lead others on this journey. You are the source of light and love, God. I am an expression of you and I am here to shine.

Energy Foundation Tracker

I ate breakfast.	■
I ate smaller healthy meals and energizing snacks.	■
I drank plenty of water.	■
I slept enough to feel energized and rested.	■
I engaged in some form of physical activity.	■
I listened to energizing music.	■
I connected with people who increase my energy.	■
I practiced my energizer breath when stressed.	■

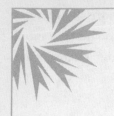

Week 3 Day 18

Lose Your Mind for 10 Minutes

"The caterpillar must surrender to the cocoon before it becomes a butterfly."

—Author Unknown

People often get intimidated when they hear the word "meditation." But, really, silent energy and meditation are one and the same. Meditation is nothing more than focusing your energy on the present moment, silencing your thoughts and your mind while maintaining an alert and focused state of openness and awareness, and cultivating a state of positive emotion. Ironically, in "mindfulness meditations," you don't want to have a mind full of thoughts but rather a mind full of "nothingness."

While meditating, you want to lose your thoughts, your thinking, and your mind so you can be one with the moment. If a thought pops into your head such as, "I wonder what I'll have for dinner tonight," you let it float in, float by, and then return to silence. It's something that is difficult to describe but easily understood when you practice it. As I stated earlier in the plan, the latest research shows that meditation strengthens our immune system, reduces stress, creates more activation in the left-prefrontal cortex (the site of our brain associated with positive emotions), and increases our happiness and energy levels. Meditation is like high-octane fuel for our mind and body. It helps you to live in the present moment, and I believe it connects you to your deeper timeless self and to the energy all around you.

While some people associate meditation with a particular Eastern religion, please understand that meditation can be practiced by people of all religions. I have helped people from all walks of life—including athletes, actors, artists, corporate executives, and moms and dads—learn how to meditate, and they all experience the benefits. Whereas a chaotic and busy life makes you feel like two people living a split existence, meditation helps to integrate your split existence into one powerful you. Instead of always thinking of the future or letting your thoughts take you into the past, meditation helps you focus your attention and energy on the "here" and "now," where life is truly lived.

So just as we can train our bodies by lifting weights, meditation is the ultimate workout for our mind. Meditation helps you build the mental and emotional muscle you need to live a happier, more positive life, and it should be part of your daily routine—after all, it takes only 10 minutes. Remember, as is true with any exercise, the more you do it, the more natural it feels, the stronger you become, and the more results you create. The lifelong habit of meditation produces profound and incredible lifelong results. After you complete this plan, I hope you make meditation one of the exercises you incorporate into your daily life. Let's begin our practice of meditations by "losing our mind" for 10 minutes today.

SCHEDULE YOUR 10 MINUTES OF MEDITATION today. What time will you take this energy break? Commit to it! Write the time of day or specific time on your calendar or PDA.

Action Steps

➤ Find a quiet place. Perhaps it's your office or bedroom or a park bench outside your office. Sit in a comfortable position.

➤ Start focusing on your breathing, inhaling through your nose and exhaling through your nose and mouth. Focus on your breath as it lifts the belly, and follow it as it lifts your diaphragm, chest, and then shoulders. Focus on your breath as you exhale and it leaves your body. Relax and let your breath get quieter and lighter.

➤ Continue to focus on your breathing. As you inhale, think of a word such as "so" or "energy" or "one" or "God" or a specific word that is meaningful to you. If you are a beach lover, you may think "beach." When exhaling think of the word "hum" or "energy" or "one" or "God."

➤ Continue breathing, silently repeating, "so, hum," or another combination of words. The "so hum" technique is one that I practice and learned from author and mind/body pioneer Deepak Chopra.

➤ As thoughts come into your mind, don't fight them. Let them flow in and flow out. Focus on your breathing and your words. This keeps your mind alert but relaxed. Continue this process for 10 minutes. You'll be amazed how fast 10 minutes pass.

➤ Write down in your journal how you feel.

Understand that if you are new to this exercise, it will feel a little awkward at first, but after a little practice, it will feel quite natural.

11th-Minute Miracle

God, today I ask you to grant me the patience to practice meditation so that I may realize the benefits of this incredible exercise. I ask you for the dedication to make meditation a routine part of my life. I ask for a calm mind so that I can connect more deeply with myself and my infinite source of energy. I ask that you allow me to use meditation to connect with you, for when I am silent, I feel your presence—and for a brief time I am tuned into the energy that powers everything. I ask that you allow me to fuel up with this energy and let it energize all the areas of my life. Let meditation help me create and share your miracles. Flow through me and let my practice of meditation be the tool that opens my pipeline to you.

Energy Foundation Tracker

I ate breakfast.	▪
I ate smaller healthy meals and energizing snacks.	▪
I drank plenty of water.	▪
I slept enough to feel energized and rested.	▪
I engaged in some form of physical activity.	▪
I listened to energizing music.	▪
I connected with people who increase my energy.	▪
I practiced my energizer breath when stressed.	▪

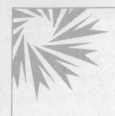

Week 3 Day 19

Let Go of Your Stress and Fear

"Ultimately we know deeply that the other side of fear is freedom"

—Marilyn Ferguson

Stress is simply the physical and emotional manifestation of our thoughts and emotions. Think of yourself as an energy pipeline, where energy flows from your head to your toes. Now realize that energy is always flowing through you. The key is how you process this energy. If your internal energy machine keeps the energy light and flowing, then you'll feel calm, healthy, energized, and peaceful. However, if your energy machine doesn't work very well because it is stressed, this can cause your energy to get thick and sludgy. This creates a blockage in your energy pipeline, which drains your energy and leads to more stress, fatigue, and poor health.

It is important to realize that our bodies require communication between our cells via electromagnetic signals or frequencies to maintain harmony, balance, and health. Each cell needs to know what all the others are doing in order for us to not fall apart. Unfortunately, stress affects this inner intelligence and harmony—it's like a radio signal jammer that affects our cells' ability to communicate with each other. This leads to disharmony and disease inside the body.

By creating a calm, powerful, and centered "energy machine" (i.e., body) that keeps your energy light and flowing, you will maintain harmony and let go of your stress. However, while letting go of stress is very helpful, it is not the complete solution. In the process of letting go of our stress, we also find a deeper layer of sludge we know as fear, which is just below the surface of stress and is the root cause of stress. Just as we don't clean a swimming pool by skimming only the leaves off the surface, we can't let go of our stress by practicing only "letting go" of stress exercises. To fully clean our energy pipeline, we must dig a little deeper and let go of the fear that gives rise to our stress.

With every stressful thought, you will find that fear is the root cause. If you are stressed about finishing a project, you will find that you fear not having enough time. Or perhaps you have a deeper fear of failure. If you are stressed about money, then you will find a fear of not being secure or provided for. If you are stressed about your job or an upcoming meeting at work, you probably will find a fear of "not being enough" or a fear that others won't approve of you. Fear is the antithesis of trust, which we will talk about next week, and fear can destroy your health and the quality of your life if left unchecked. Just as we let go of our stress earlier, we must let go of our fear to lose the negative energy that slows us down and holds us back.

When making the decision to let go of fear, remember the FEAR acronym many of us have seen before. False Evidence Appearing Real. While your fear may seem so powerful and scary if you place your attention on it and look right directly into it, you realize fear is just an illusion. Fear is the result of our thoughts created by the ego. It helps us control, fight, separate, dominate, run, and survive—but it will not help us relax, be happy, get calm, and thrive. To thrive, we must let go of our fear, which we will do today and replace it with trust, which we will do next week. So today do a double dose of letting go by letting go of your stress and fear. To let go of your stress and fear and become a flowing energy pipeline, practice the following letting go exercise.

SCHEDULE YOUR 10 MINUTES: Decide what time of day you will practice your letting go exercises. Morning? Lunch? Evening? Make an appointment with yourself now.

Action Steps

➤ First identify the stress you are feeling. Perhaps you are stressed about your job or paying bills. Perhaps you are stressed that you have a meeting this afternoon and you can't find a babysitter for your children. Perhaps you are stressed about finishing a project. Or maybe you are stressed about meeting new people at a party or work function. Write down your stresses below. Identifying your stresses will help you release them. Complete the following sentences.

I am stressed that _____.

I am stressed about _____

because _____.

My main stresses are _____.

➤ Now take several deep breaths, inhaling for three seconds and exhaling for three seconds. Think about the stress that is causing you pain and discomfort. Don't fight it. Accept that you are currently holding on to it.

➤ Now say the following: "I understand the stresses that I am feeling and I choose to let them go. They are feelings and I don't have to hold on to them. I let go of all my stresses."

➤ Then take a deep cleansing breath, making a fist with both hands, and act as if you are holding on to all the fear and stress inside you. Then exhale forcefully as you open your hands and release your arms out and away from your body. Your arms should end up being wide open, as if you were a child saying, "The fish was this big." You should feel all your tension released.

I call this a cleansing breath. While exhaling, imagine yourself breathing out all the stress, fear, and resistance inside you.

➤ After this breath, say, "I let go of my fear and stress. I choose not to have it. I let it go."

➤ Repeat the last two steps five times as you focus your mind and your thoughts on letting go.

➤ Now use those steps to let go of each specific stress individually. For example, if you wrote in the exercise above that you were stressed about not having enough time to finish a project, you might say, "I let go of this stress about finishing my project. I choose not to have it. I let it go." Then you might say, "I have all the time I need to do everything I need to do."

Now let's let go of your fears.

➤ First identify your fears. What are your common fears? Do you fear not having enough money? Failure? Losing your job? Flying? Not finding the right person? Getting old? Gaining weight?

➤ Complete the following sentences.

My number one fear is _____.

I fear that _____.

I am fearful of _____.

My fear is that _____.

➤ Now just as you let go of your stress, it's time to let go of your fear. Take several deep breaths, inhaling for three seconds and exhaling for three seconds. Think about the fear that is causing you pain and discomfort. Don't fight it. Accept that you are currently holding on to it.

➤ Now say the following: "I understand the fear that I am feeling and I choose to let it go. Fear is just a feeling and I don't have to hold on to it. I let go of all my fears."

➤ Then take a deep cleansing breath, making a fist with both hands, and act as if you are holding on to all the fear inside you. Then exhale forcefully as you open your hands and release your arms out and away from your body. While exhaling, imagine yourself breathing out all the fear and resistance inside you.

➤ After this breath, say, "I let go of my fear. I choose not to have it. I let it go."

➤ Repeat the last two steps five times as you focus your mind and your thoughts on letting go.

➤ Now use these steps to let go of each specific fear individually. For example, if you wrote in the exercise above that you were fearful that you won't have enough money to live the life you want, you might say, "I let go of my fear about money. I choose not to have it. I let it go." Then you might say, "I have all the money I need to do everything I need to do."

➤ Once you have finished letting go of each fear, take a few deep breaths. Close your eyes and imagine that your energy pipeline is a lot clearer than it was. Visualize yourself on a boat dock and imagine that all your fears are floating away.

➤ Write down in your journal how you feel.

➤ Practice this exercise whenever you feel stressed and fearful.

11th Minute Miracle

I surrender my stress and fear to you, God. I give them to you. I don't want them. I surrender this resistance that I feel. I release it so that I can flow. I let it go so I can connect to you, God. God, please give me the strength to let go of what holds me back. Help me clear this negative energy from my mind and body. Make me an instrument of your peace and calm. Make me a conduit for your flowing positive energy. Allow me to feel lighter, happier, and freer. Send me a miracle, God. I am ready for a miracle.

Energy Foundation Tracker

I ate breakfast.	■
I ate smaller healthy meals and energizing snacks.	■
I drank plenty of water.	■
I slept enough to feel energized and rested.	■
I engaged in some form of physical activity.	■
I listened to energizing music.	■
I connected with people who increase my energy.	■
I practiced my energizer breath when stressed.	■

Forgive and Experience the Ultimate Weight Loss

"Holding on to resentment and anger is like grasping a hot coal with the intent of throwing it at someone else. You are the one who gets burned."

—Buddha

There is a horse farmer near my house in northeast Florida who shares his own profound quotes by posting signs on his property near the highway for thousands of drivers to see on the way to and from work. This past week he posted a sign that said, FORGIVENESS IS THE ULTIMATE WEIGHT LOSS. While yesterday's 10-minute exercises helped you let go of your fear and stress, the real heavy energy starts to come off when you make the decision to let go of your resentment, pain, and anger—and the way to do this is to forgive.

Consider forgiveness as one of the key components of a negative energy diet. When you forgive, you release emotional fat. You let go of the heavy energy that weighs you down. You let go of the past, which doesn't have to be a part of your future. You forgive yourself for your past indiscretions. You forgive people who have hurt you. You forgive your family for the mistakes they made when raising you. You forgive yourself for not being perfect. You forgive life for not being what you expected it to be. Whereas stress represents the surface level of sludge that clogs our energy pipeline, and fear resides below stress, anger and resentment reside even farther below fear. To let go, we must go within a little deeper. Like an excavator we must break through the surface and connect with our energy blocks so we can clear them out. Forgiveness is the ultimate tool to accomplish this task. When you forgive, you will release what needs to be excavated and experience the ultimate negative energy weight loss.

SCHEDULE YOUR 10 MINUTES: Decide what time of day you will practice your letting go exercises. Morning? Lunch? Evening? Make an appointment with yourself now.

Action Steps

➤ Identify what percentage of your energy you spend living in the past, thinking negative thoughts, and feeling angry or resentful about those who have hurt you. Ten percent? Fifty percent? Eighty percent? Make a conscious choice right now to invest more of your energy in the present moment.

➤ Make a list of what anger and/or resentment is holding you back. Perhaps it's a boss who fired you. Perhaps it's something your spouse did. Perhaps it's something you did to yourself or someone else. Maybe it's a traumatic event such as verbal or physical abuse. Write down your anger and resentments now in your journal.

➤ Complete the following sentences

I forgive _____ for _____.
              (whom)   (doing what)

I forgive myself for _____.

➤ I let go of the pain and resentment I feel when I think about _____.
                                                              (what event)

because it happened in the past and the past is not who I am. Today I invest my energy here and now. I accept what happened. I acknowledge what happened. But I let go of it and I allow myself to be free of the pain it has caused me.

➤ Read the three sentences above aloud five times as you put your hands on your heart. As you say each sentence, see the person that you are forgiving. If you are forgiving yourself, look in the mirror. Imagine that as you are forgiving, you are directing positive energy through your hands and into your heart, healing it in the process.

➤ Repeat the above steps if there are more people and events you need to let go of and forgive.

➤ Now write a letter of forgiveness. Write it to yourself (if you are forgiving yourself) or to someone who you want to forgive. Realize that you are not writing this letter for them. You don't have to send it. You are writing it for yourself. You are writing it for your benefit. You are writing it to let go and heal. It's a choice between living and dying each day. Even the Central Park jogger chose to forgive her attackers who left her for dead because she said she wanted to live instead of die each day. When we forgive, we choose to live. When we hold on to anger and resentment, we choose to let our life wilt away. Write your letter now. Start with "I forgive . . ."

➤ Realize that forgiveness is not easy. If this is a difficult exercise for you, then don't rush it. Awareness is the first step. Go as far as you can with this exercise. You can come back and excavate further another day. Do what you feel comfortable with and revisit this exercise again.

11th-Minute Miracle

Forgive me, God. Forgive me for my faults. Forgive me for holding on to my anger and resentment all these years. Forgive me for being selfish at different times in my life. Forgive me for ignoring and not trusting you, God. Today I make a commitment to you that I will continue to learn and grow and improve. I forgive others as part of this growth and, most important, I forgive myself. I pray that you will help me through this forgiveness process, God. It is not easy, but in your strength I can do it. I pray for the strength to let go of the pain and anger inside me. I pray that you will flow through me as I heal my past, improve my present, and create hope for my future. I let go of my past, God. It is not who I am, and it is not who I am going to be. I commit to creating my future with you, God—one miracle at a time.

Energy Foundation Tracker

I ate breakfast.	▨
I ate smaller healthy meals and energizing snacks.	▨
I drank plenty of water.	▨
I slept enough to feel energized and rested.	▨
I engaged in some form of physical activity.	▨
I listened to energizing music.	▨
I connected with people who increase my energy.	▨
I practiced my energizer breath when stressed.	▨

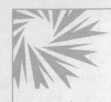

Ditch Your Ego

When we dig past stress and fear and go below anger and resentment, we get to the ultimate source of all pain, unhappiness, stress, and human sludge. The *ego*. The ego wants and needs control, power, love, approval, and security. The ego also has a tremendous desire to be separate. The ego creates a me vs. you attitude. It causes you to crave money as a means of security. It causes power struggles in corporations and marriages and leads to wars between countries. It causes you to be a perfectionist to gain approval from others. It makes you crave recognition from coworkers and love from your partner. The ego makes you feel anxious and uptight when things don't go as planned. It causes you to feel separate from the people closest to you, and it clogs up the pipeline between you and your higher power and greater source of energy.

Ego stands for Edging God Out. Imagine with me for a moment that you and your higher power, or "source," are connected by an energy pipeline. You came from this source and are an expression of this source, so you are always connected to it. However, your ego causes you to think and feel as if you are separate from your source and separate from others. It makes you think you are in control instead of God. It tells you a lie that you can create security when "acts of God" teach you that security is an illusion. Anyone who has lived through a hurricane knows this. The ego keeps you busy so you don't make time to connect with your source, and when you take time to connect, it creates the sludge that blocks this connection between you and your higher power. While you are always connected to your source, the ego stops the flow of energy meant for you. All the resistance that you feel is a result of the ego-producing sludge that separates you from your source. Like a child who feels uncomfortable because she misses her parents, you are feeling discomfort because you are not connected with your source.

If you could get rid of your ego, you would always feel connected. You wouldn't know fear. You would always feel at peace, and you would never experience doubt. Without an ego you would always be one with your source and possess the same abundance and positive flowing energy. But, unfortunately, we do have an ego and it does not go away easily. As Wayne Dyer jokes, it's not like you can get an ego-ectomy. But thankfully you can do exercises that serve as your Liquid Ego Drano that will help you let go of the ego and create a more powerful connection to your source. With each letting go exercise, you release more and more of your energy blockage. This leads to greater peace, happiness, and abundance.

SCHEDULE YOUR 10 MINUTES: Decide what time of day you will practice your letting go exercises. Morning? Lunch? Evening? Make an appointment with yourself now.

Action Steps

➤ Take a deep cleansing breath, just as we learned how to do earlier this week. Make a fist with both hands, then exhale forcefully as you open your hands and release your arms out and away from your body. Your arms should end up being wide open, and you should feel all your tension released. While exhaling, imagine yourself breathing out all the stress, fear, and resistance inside you.

➤ Then say the following sentences. After each sentence take a cleansing breath, visualizing yourself releasing your energy blockage and flowing with positive energy.

"I let go of my ego that wants control. I am not in control. I let go of my need for control. I surrender it. I trust that everything happens for a reason."

[Cleansing breath]

"I let go of my ego that wants security. Security is an illusion. I let go of my need for security. I surrender it. I trust that everything happens for a reason."

[Cleansing breath]

"I let go of my ego that wants love. I let go of my need for love. I am an abundant source of love. I am an infinite expression of love."

[Cleansing breath]

"I let go of my ego that wants approval. All I need to do is shine my light, my joy, my gifts, and my happiness."

[Cleansing breath]

"I let go of my ego that wants to be separate. I am one with everyone and everything in the universe."

[Cleansing breath]

➤ Repeat the sentences above until your 10 minutes are up. Feel free to say each sentence several times before moving on to the next sentence. **Hint:** Feel free to do this exercise while you are walking. I do this exercise during my daily walk.

➤ Describe how you feel after this exercise and write it down in your journal.

11th-Minute Miracle

I let go of my ego that stops me from connecting to you, God. I let go of my ego that wants control. I surrender to you, God. Use me for your purpose and guide me toward my purpose. Flow through me. I let go of my ego that wants security. Today I ask you to be my security adviser, God. I trust in you. I know that I am secure only in your energy and strength. I trust that everything happens for a reason, and I trust that every problem has a lesson plan with it. I trust that you will show me the way and guide me toward my highest purpose and greatest good. I let it go so miracles can flow. I am ready for a miracle, God. Send me a miracle when the time is right.

Energy Foundation Tracker

I ate breakfast.	▨
I ate smaller healthy meals and energizing snacks.	▨
I drank plenty of water.	▨
I slept enough to feel energized and rested.	▨
I engaged in some form of physical activity.	▨
I listened to energizing music.	▨
I connected with people who increase my energy.	▨
I practiced my energizer breath when stressed.	▨

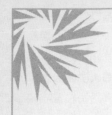

Week 3

Evaluation— Where Are You Now?

You've completed the third week of the plan. You are three-fourths of the way there. So how was it? Do you feel more alive, more focused, more positive? Complete the following scales, and let me know how you are doing. I would love to hear from you. E-mail me at jon@jongordon.com. Also visit me at www.jongordon.com to receive an energy boost for the final week of the plan.

Negative Energy–Positive Energy Scale

| 1 | 2 | 3 | 4 | 5 | 6 | 7 | 8 | 9 | 1 0 |

Negative   Positive

Sad-Happy Scale

| 1 | 2 | 3 | 4 | 5 | 6 | 7 | 8 | 9 | 1 0 |

Sad   Happy

Stressed Scale

| 1 | 2 | 3 | 4 | 5 | 6 | 7 | 8 | 9 | 1 0 |

Stressed   Relaxed

Focused Scale

1	2	3	4	5	6	7	8	9	1 0

Scattered   Focused

Fear-Trust Scale

1	2	3	4	5	6	7	8	9	1 0

Fear   Trust

Overall Energy Scale

1	2	3	4	5	6	7	8	9	1 0

Low   High

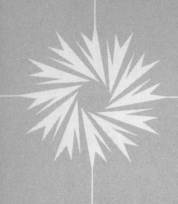

Chapter 8

The 10-Minute-a-Day Plan— Week 4

Add 10 Minutes of Spiritual Energy to Your Day

There are those who say life is like a sprint or a marathon. I say it often feels like a sprint combined with a boxing match, because not only are we running but we're also getting hit along the way. Every day we face challenges and obstacles that feel like we're getting battered with left jabs and right hooks. Sure we have goals, but many folks could care less about our goals. We have dreams that others can't see. We have a vision that only plays in our mind . . . no one else's. We have hopes for our relationships, our families, our careers. But then, *bam. Whack. Bam.* We're hit again, and we lose our footing.

Negative comments from relatives, energy vampires at work, tax bills, rejections, challenging customers, difficult children, self-doubt, and problematic relationships all take their toll on us. Now more than ever, it is imperative to build our mental, emotional, and spiritual muscle to overcome life's adversity. Just as a boxer needs to train his body to compete, we need to train our minds to develop the mental, emotional, and spiritual strength to withstand the barrage that life can often bring.

In the Academy Award–winning movie *Million Dollar Baby*, Maggie had a vision for her life. She knew with the right training she could be a champion. She received that training and the crowds cheered her. So I ask you, what could you accomplish with the right training to overcome the adversity, the challenges, and the negativity in your life? What would you achieve if self-doubt didn't stop the flow of positive energy in your life? We'll never be able to change others—only they can change themselves. And we'll never have a challenge-free life. What we must do is develop and train ourselves. We must reach a point where our positive energy, vision, enthusiasm, and trust are greater than anyone's negativity or any one challenging event. Our certainty must become greater than their doubt.

So how do we do this? We start by fueling our life with spiritual energy. As Einstein said, we bring a new awareness, a new perspective, and a higher level of thinking to deal with life's daily challenges and struggles. We fill our life and our thinking with spiritual energy in the form of trust and love—the most powerful sources of energy in the universe. Whereas gas is expensive and in short supply these days, trust and love are infinite . . . and so priceless they are free. Whereas gas makes cars move, spiritual energy moves everything in the universe, including you.

When I think of spiritual energy, I picture a water balloon in the middle of an ocean. We are the water in the balloon, and the ocean is the sea of energy in which we live. The rubber of the balloon separates us from the ocean. It keeps us from our source. The rubber represents the ego and lower vibration thoughts and emotions. The more stress, fear, anger, resentment, doubt, and pain you feel the thicker the rubber becomes. However, when we find silence and live with positive energy, the rubber dissolves. That's why we feel more at peace when we meditate, play, and pray. And when we trust and love, the rubber evaporates. The separation between you and me and you and your higher power disappears. Through trust and love we become one with our source and we become one with all the power, all the energy, and all the abundance that exist. Like standing at the ultimate gas station we fuel up with spiritual energy, and this provides us with high-octane fuel for everyday life.

Since trust and love are so important, the next question is, How do we create a life filled with more trust and love? We create it by exercising and building our spiritual muscles. Trust and love don't just occur by osmosis. With our gift of free will, we must make the decision to trust and love. It is a choice. We must build and cultivate trust and love in ourselves and believe in a bigger plan for our life.

It is a choice I know well. A few years ago when I was miserable with my life—taking a daily beating from stress and fear—I finally made the decision to trust and love. I came up with a mantra, and I started saying it throughout the day every day. In fact, I still say this daily: "I trust that great things are happening today and I am a powerful expression of love." I find the less I fear and the more I trust and love, the more my life flows. Try it and see for yourself. The more you do this exercise, the more automatic and stronger the response becomes.

When you are faced with a fearful or stressful situation, don't let fear hijack your thoughts and mind. Instead, flex your spiritual muscles and let love dominate your thought process. Instead of thinking, "What are we going to do, this is bad, I can't handle this, it's hopeless, why me, what's going to happen tomorrow," you will trust and say, "Calm down, relax, everything is going to work out, it always does, I can handle it, and I trust that great things are happening." Building your spiritual muscles will help you make better decisions at work and at home. It will help you reduce stress. You will flow instead of fight each day. And, most important, your trust and faith will energize you to take on each day, each challenge, and each situation one trusting and loving belief at a time. Trust that great things are happening and they will.

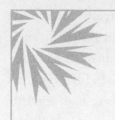

Replace Fear
with Trust

"Fear knocked at the door. Trust answered
and no one was there."

—Anonymous

When you let go of your stress, fear, and ego last week, you released
the negative heavy energy inside you and helped clear your energy
pipeline. This process is enhanced ever further when you replace fear
with trust. Think of trust as high-octane spiritual energy that, when
poured down your energy pipeline, prevents sludge from accumulat-
ing and clears out your stress, fear, and negative energy.

Trust is the antidote to fear and the ego's archenemy. Where there
is trust, fear cannot survive. Whereas the ego creates a lower, heavier
vibration within our energy field, trust brings a lighter, higher vibration to our mental, physical, emotional, and spiritual energy. It
changes our energy from resistance to acceptance—from struggle to
flow. Where fear cuts off the flow of energy into your life, trust opens
the door to abundance, limitless possibilities, and a bigger plan for
your life.

As I have studied people throughout my life, I have always been
amazed that for the people who always stay calm and relaxed during
difficult times everything always seems to work out—as if they lived
a charmed existence. Whereas the people who stress to the max and
live a life of fear always find themselves in one crisis and struggle after another. As a person who lived one struggle after another, I
would look upon the "charmed" people with awe and anger at the
same time. *Why couldn't I have been born like that?* I wondered.

Why them and not me? But then I discovered the truth. I found research that showed people aren't *born* charmed, but rather through trust they *create* a charmed existence. A British study looked at four hundred people who supposedly lived "charmed lives." To the outside world these people had it all—nothing bad ever happened to them. What researchers found was that it wasn't that bad things didn't happen to them, but rather that, when bad fortune struck, they turned it into good. These supposedly charmed people acted upon opportunities, paid attention to gut feelings, expected good fortune, and turned bad into good. In other words, they trusted and they fueled their life with trust.

We all know that we can never stop bad things from happening. It's part of our human drama to experience suffering and bliss, happiness and sadness, defeat and victory, love and loss. And while I don't claim it is easy and I realize that many people have suffered much more than me, I know there is tremendous power and peace in living with trust. The road through challenges, adversity, and negative events is paved with a "great things are happening" philosophy. While at the time we may not see the lesson or the bigger plan, with trust and faith we must maintain that all is good and all will lead to good. A job loss today leads to a dream job tomorrow. A mistake turns into career growth and a promotion. The betrayal that would have destroyed us makes us stronger and happier. The failed business deal is transformed into knowledge and a bigger and better deal a year from now. Even a tragedy brings us closer to the ones we love.

When I discovered the power of trust in my life, I learned that while I was born with a fearful and anxious disposition, I could develop trust and learn to overcome fear. While my first instinct is always fear, I have learned to replace this fear with trust. I repeatedly practiced on a daily basis the exercise I am about to share with you, and over time I found my trust growing stronger and my ability to handle life's setbacks and obstacles improving. Like brushing my teeth, trust became a habit—and I still work at it. It wasn't easy.

Trust, as you know, is hard to achieve. When you are faced with financial difficulties, job problems, relationship issues, and everyday life stresses, it's quite difficult to trust that "everything is going to be okay." But that's what makes this 10-minute exercise so important. You don't have to wait until you are in the middle of a crisis to develop trust. You can prepare now and the trust you develop today will serve you tomorrow. The key with this exercise is to help you shift your mind from fear to trust. It won't feel natural at first, but over time trust will become your predominant response.

SCHEDULE YOUR 10 MINUTES: Decide what time of day you will practice your trust exercises. Morning? Lunch? Evening? Make an appointment with yourself now.

Action Steps

➤ Write down your list of fears. What are you stressed about? What worries you on a daily basis? Perhaps you are worried about losing your job or paying your bills. Perhaps you are fearful that you won't lose weight. Perhaps you are scared that you won't achieve a particular goal. Write down your worries and fears below or in your journal.

I am worried that _____.

I am fearful that _____.

I'm scared that _____.

I'm stressed about _____ because _____.

I'm worried that_____.

➤ Now, realize that fear serves no purpose. It is useless to spend energy being fearful about the things you can't control. Fear stops the flow of positive energy into your life. Understand that all you can do is trust because ultimately you are not in control. This doesn't mean you don't take action, but, rather, you trust that your positive actions will serve your highest purpose.

➤ Complete the following sentences as you think about your list of fears and worries listed above.

> ➤ I am not worried about _____because whatever is going to happen will happen, and I'm not in control. I pray for guidance. I pray that I will find my purpose and my purpose will find me.
> ➤ I'm not going to be stressed about_____ because there is plenty of time to do everything I need to do. There is always enough time.
> ➤ I'm not angry about _____because I believe that everything happens for a reason. I'm just going to work hard and trust that everything will work out fine. I trust that my life will unfold the way it is supposed to, and even if something doesn't happen the way I want it to, I know it's because there is a bigger plan for me.
> ➤ I trust that great things *are* happening every day. Great things *are* happening every day. I realize that my fear regarding _____is teaching me a lesson that I need to trust that_____.

➤ Read each sentence aloud as you contemplate the meaning of what you are saying.

➤ Repeat the sentences above three times. As you say each sentence, realize that each sentence represents the truth. Sure, your negative thoughts might say, "Yeah, right." Allow these thoughts to come in and let them go. They represent your fighting ego that wants to hold onto control. Your ego doesn't want you to trust. Don't let your ego win. Believe in something bigger than yourself. Trust that what looks bleak today will shine tomorrow. Practice trust and see for yourself.

➤ Describe how you feel after this exercise and write it in your journal.

11th-Minute Miracle

It's so hard to trust when nothing is going right. I often feel as if my life is spinning out of control. So I ask you to help me see beyond my current challenges. Help me to recognize that problems only make me stronger. Give me the strength to overcome my difficulties and challenges. Help me have the perspective that everything will work out. Help me believe that everything happens for a reason. And as I ask for help, God, I also know it's up to me. So I commit to you that I will trust. I trust that you will guide me. I trust that you wouldn't bring me to a certain situation if you wouldn't see me through it. I trust that everything will work out the way it is supposed to. I trust that you have a bigger plan in store for me. I trust that my life is going in the right direction. I trust.

Energy Foundation Tracker

I ate breakfast.	▪
I ate smaller healthy meals and energizing snacks.	▪
I drank plenty of water.	▪

I slept enough to feel energized and rested.

I engaged in some form of physical activity.

I listened to energizing music.

I connected with people who increase my energy.

I practiced my energizer breath when stressed.

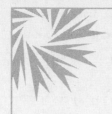

Believe That Everything Happens for a Reason

> "I complained to God when my foundation was shaking, only to discover that it was God who was shaking it."
>
> —Charles Weston

The ultimate choice we face every moment of every day is between trust and fear. If you are not yet convinced of the power of trust, I want to ask you to think about a difficult time in your life. Perhaps it's a bad breakup or an unhappy marriage. Perhaps it's a time when you were fired or cut from a sports team. Or perhaps it was when you lost a business deal or made a big mistake. Now I want to ask you if you grew stronger from this experience. Did it make you a better person? Ninety percent of the people to whom I ask these questions answer "yes."

Richard Bach said, "Every problem has a gift for you in its hands," and it appears every struggle makes you a better and stronger person. We don't know why things happen to us, and we can't control them. But what we can do is trust that the problems we are facing today will make us stronger tomorrow. Consider a Gallup poll in which they asked participants to identify the worst thing and the best thing that ever happened to them. Amazingly, researchers found an 80 percent correlation between the worst and best thing. The worst thing somehow leads to the best thing. The understanding of this research is beyond our comprehension and leads to only one conclusion. Trust. We can't control what happens to us. But we can control whether we fear or trust. As I write this, I want you to know that I speak not only as a teacher and researcher but as someone who has lived this.

It seems like only yesterday that I was brought to my knees for the first time. I was about to open my own restaurant. I also had a job with a company that was going downhill. It was during the dot.com bust, and our bubble was getting ready to burst. I had just read the book *Who Moved My Cheese?*, and this company's cheese did not smell good. My goal was to keep my job until my restaurant made a profit. Once the restaurant was profitable, I planned to start my real passion—writing and speaking. My wife and I were taking a big risk. Every dollar we owned was invested in the restaurant. We even mortgaged our home to come up with the start-up funds.

My plan was coming together until, well, let's just say God had other plans. A week before my restaurant was set to open, I got the call from my boss. The company was downsizing. Channeling Donald Trump, he said, "Jon, you're fired." I got off the phone. My face turned pale white. My heart started to race. What about my family? What about health insurance for my wife and two children? What if the restaurant doesn't make it? What about my mortgage? We had only two months of savings in the bank. They gave me only two weeks' severance pay. Now I had to go face my wife and tell her I was fired. Talk about a humbling experience—to tell the one you love that you have failed. That your future is in serious doubt. That you may be going bankrupt. That you may have to move. She consoled me, but I was crumbling. I went upstairs to my home office—alone, scared, and crying. For the first time in my life I was brought to my knees. I was broken. For the first time in my life Mr. Control Freak was not in control. Mr. I Can Do It Myself couldn't do it alone. I almost had a breakdown, but it was the best thing that ever happened to me.

I call it my Jerry Maguire moment. *Jerry Maguire* is one of my favorite movies because Jerry had to lose everything to become the person he was meant to be. Sometimes a person has to lose a goal to find their destiny. I looked up to the heavens, and for the first time in my life, I surrendered. I said, "Help me, God. Help me help you. Help meeeeeeeee, help youuuuuuu. Provide for me and my family, and I will do your work. I will do everything I can to make a difference in the world." At that moment this incredible feeling of peace came over me, and I was filled with a belief that everything happens for a reason. I realized that I lost my job for a reason, and I needed to trust that everything would work out. I was being taught a lesson. The next day, and every day, I marketed the restaurant 1000 percent. It's amazing what you'll do when your family's future is on the line. We broke even the first, second, third, and fourth week. We weren't losing money but weren't making it either. Now my wife and I had only one month of savings. I kept on marketing and trusting that everything would work out.

My wife was getting her résumé together when I received a call out of the blue from a friend in Atlanta. He said he just spoke with a company in my city that wanted to learn about wireless software. I met with this company, and amazingly they agreed to pay me $13,000 for just six weeks of consulting. You bet I did the touchdown dance when I came home. My wife said, "Jon, don't you see it, we are being carried." Over the next few months I kept on repeating the sentence, "Everything happens for a reason," and as the last dime ran out of our bank account, our restaurant made its first profit. It was like clockwork. The sign was clear. Trust and let the abundance flow. Several months later, after a few continuous profitable months, I started writing and speaking, and several years later you are now reading this book.

I became a new person after this experience, and my hope is that after reading this, you will also make the decision to trust and believe that everything happens for a reason. Although I can't promise that you won't face hardships, illnesses, or financial difficulties, I can promise that trust will help you overcome them. I have learned that in order to change a situation, you must change the energy you project. When you trust, you become a conduit for abundance, supportive people, money, and positive energy that fearful energy blocks but trusting energy accepts. You become a magnet for the impossible. You become a walking miracle. You don't know why things happen, but you realize there is a bigger plan. And while you can't comprehend it now, you know that everything happens for a reason and that eventually the reason will be revealed to you. The hardest thing in the world is to let go of our control and to trust, but take it from someone who knows—when we trust, let go, and flow, magical things happen. I trust and hope you will experience this magic for yourself by trying the following exercise to strengthen your trust muscles.

SCHEDULE YOUR 10 MINUTES: Decide what time of day you will practice your trust exercises. Morning? Lunch? Evening? Make an appointment with yourself now.

Action Steps

➤ As if you were describing your life to a reporter, write down the struggles, obstacles, challenges, or problems you are currently experiencing in your life. Share with the reporter a picture of your life. Describe this picture in your journal, as if you were describing a movie.

➤ Then consider the lessons you could be learning from this movie of your life. For each problem or struggle, ask, "What is the lesson here?" If an answer doesn't come to you right away, that's okay. Give it a few minutes. If no answers come to you, that's fine. Simply move on to the next step. However, if you understand your lessons, write them down in your journal.

➤ Now imagine your life five or ten years into the future. Visualize yourself as a calmer, happier, more trusting person. Think about what two or three different versions of your life may look like. Think of three different scenarios that could happen if you could dissolve the obstacles you currently face. Think about the job you have. Visualize the success and happiness you enjoy. Consider what your life would be like if everything worked out. Visualize your life if trust allowed you to flow with abundance. Now describe these different lives to a reporter by writing them in your journal.

Possible Life 1

Possible Life 2

Possible Life 3

➤ Consider these two or three possible lives. Take a few minutes and trust that they are possible for you. Perhaps not every aspect of each life but maybe a combination of them or some aspects of them.

➤ Realize that this exercise shifted your mind-set to think about what is possible. What could be—what might happen. This mental shift is available to you any time you are stuck in a life predicament. Remember when you are feeling down, hope and trust float.

➤ Write down in your journal how you feel after this exercise.

11th-Minute Miracle

Open my eyes to the miracles all around me, God. Widen my ears so I can hear miraculous conversations. Enlarge my trust so I can envision a bigger plan and miracle that is meant for me. I am ready to take a leap of faith, God. I understand that they don't call it a leap of fear for a reason. They call it a leap of faith, and I am ready to fuel up with trust and take my leap today. Today I give you my fear and I accept trust. Today I rise up above the muck and goo in my life and I see the possibilities and hope that exists all around me. I realize how fear has limited me all these years, and today I commit to breaking free—to live the life I was born to live. I am ready to embrace trust as a mind-set, a philosophy, and a way of life. I am ready to energize my life with the power of trust.

Energy Foundation Tracker

I ate breakfast.	▪
I ate smaller healthy meals and energizing snacks.	▪
I drank plenty of water.	▪
I slept enough to feel energized and rested.	▪
I engaged in some form of physical activity.	▪
I listened to energizing music.	▪
I connected with people who increase my energy.	▪
I practiced my energizer breath when stressed.	▪

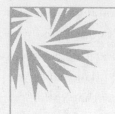

Week 4 Day 24

Take a Walk of Trust and Tap into the Energy Flow

"When you have learned how to decide with God, all decisions become as easy and as right as breathing. There is no effort and you will be led as gently as if you were being carried down a quiet path in summer."

—*A Course in Miracles*

One of my favorite ways to build my spiritual muscles is to take a walk of trust. While I walk, I cultivate a mental, emotional, and spiritual state of trust that fuels my day and my life. I have a feeling this will be one of your favorite exercises in this plan, and my hope is that while you are walking, you will picture the analogy I am about to share with you:

Consider a flowing river that represents the river of life. Now consider an iceberg in the middle of the river. Ice, as we know, is a slower vibration form of water and energy. Ice is condensed and restricted, whereas water flows freely. Steam would be considered an even higher vibration form of water. Realize that when you are living in stress and fear, you are like the iceberg in the middle of the river. All the abundance of the river is flowing toward you, but because you are frozen in a state of lower vibration, the river of life flows over you and around you but not with you. Fear causes you to resist the flow of life, while all the people who trust flow with the river. You miss all the abundance and flow that is available to you, and as you look around, you see others flowing with this abundance while you struggle, barely moving an inch at a time. You don't understand why this is happening and say things like, "Why do great things always happen to them but not me?" But now you realize it is because you are the iceberg in the flow of abundance—and now that you know this, you can change.

Understand that when you trust, you raise your vibration and you melt your iceberg. Instead of being separate from the river, you become one with the river and flow with it. You become one with all the joy, happiness, love, and abundance the river has to offer. Your frequency becomes tuned into it, and like a river that runs into the ocean you become one with your source. Trust allows you to connect with all the possibilities, all the opportunities, all the abundance that is possible for you. Instead of feeling stuck, trust allows you to tap into all the positive flowing energy that is all around you. You simply have to do the trust exercises to melt your iceberg, raise your energy vibration, and tap into the flow. To make these trust exercises even more energizing, I encourage you to practice them while taking a 10-minute walk. Call this walk your trust walk, and let it energize you mentally, physically, emotionally, and spiritually.

SCHEDULE YOUR 10 MINUTES: Decide what time of day you will practice your trust walk. Morning? Lunch? Evening? Make an appointment with yourself now.

Action Steps

➤ While walking, complete the following sentences.

I have faith that _____.

I trust that_____.

I believe that _____will

work out because everything happens for a reason.

> Read each sentence aloud. While you are saying each sentence, focus on your breathing and imagine yourself breathing in trust and letting go of fear. Visualize yourself connecting with the flow of the river with each breath.

> Continue saying these sentences for 10 minutes while you walk. When a fear-provoking event occurs today, use this time to practice your trust response. **Hint:** If you are unable to walk for any reason, then simply practice this exercise while riding a stationary bike, practicing yoga, stretching, walking in a pool, or sitting in a chair. Of course, consult your doctor before beginning any exercise routine.

> Write down in your journal how you feel after this exercise.

11th-Minute Miracle

I pray for the commitment, dedication, and strength to melt my iceberg and flow within your amazing abundance, God. I pray for the awareness to know when I am living in fear and for the ability to shift my energy into trust. I am ready to become one with the flow of life. Help me to repel the force of fear that tries to hold me back. Allow me to see what fear is, God—simply the absence of you in my life. I know when I trust in you, my fear can't take hold. I know fear is powerless when I trust in you. I trust that you will guide me. I trust that you will challenge me. I trust that you have a plan for me. I trust that when things aren't going the way I want them to, there is a reason. I trust that every problem makes me stronger and every difficult experience is a lesson. I trust that you will show me the way. Allow me to flow with you. I am ready for the ride.

Energy Foundation Tracker

I ate breakfast.	▦
I ate smaller healthy meals and energizing snacks.	▦
I drank plenty of water.	▦
I slept enough to feel energized and rested.	▦
I engaged in some form of physical activity.	▦
I listened to energizing music.	▦
I connected with people who increase my energy.	▦
I practiced my energizer breath when stressed.	▦

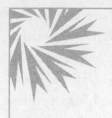

Week 4 Day 25

Cultivate Love with a Heart Walk

"As you continue to send out love, the energy returns to you in a regenerating spiral. . . . As love accumulates, it keeps your system in balance and harmony. Love is the tool, and more love is the end product."

—Sara Paddison
Hidden Power of the Heart

In addition to building our trust muscles, we must also build our love muscle, the heart. The heart, as we all know, is where we feel and express love. That's why we say, "I love them with all my heart" and "I am heartbroken because we split up" or "My heart is filled with love." But this is not just warm and fuzzy stuff that sells greeting cards and heart-shaped chocolates on Valentine's Day. The latest research in neurocardiology by the Institute of HeartMath (IHM) at www.heartmath.org demonstrates that the heart is much more than a muscle that pumps blood through our body. It is an energy pump that projects the energy of love to every cell in our body and outward. Science is now telling us what we have always intuitively known—that the heart is where we cultivate, give, and receive love.

IHM's research also demonstrates that when you cultivate feelings of love and appreciation, you create a more coherent heart rhythm—which is a sign of less stress, good health, and emotional balance. This coherent rhythm creates an organized electromagnetic field around the heart and throughout the body, which fosters better communication among your one hundred trillion energy-vibrating cells, increased mental clarity, greater energy, and improved health.

By creating a coherent heart rhythm, you create an energized heart and a harmonious mind and body. By fueling up with the spiritual energy of love, you improve every facet of your life. Like an athlete who is in the zone, you become physically and mentally energized while your focus stays relaxed, clear, and centered. You are energized and yet calm at the same time. IHM has shown that the heart is our power center and that it is the seat of our emotional and spiritual power. When you cultivate a powerful emotional and spiritual state such as the feeling of love, you supercharge your emotional energy. Combine this 10-minute emotional boost of energy with the physical and mental benefits of exercise and you exponentially increase your energy tenfold. By taking a 10-minute heart walk, you will build more love muscle that helps you develop the mental, spiritual, and emotional strength to overcomes life's daily challenges. I like to practice HeartMath's technique called Quick Coherence® while I walk. It helps me build my coherence at a time when I'm not distracted. As I say to many of my clients, including athletes and executives, while it may sound hokey to talk about love in the business or sports world, I must talk about it because coherence is love. In whatever endeavor you pursue in life, when you cultivate feelings of love, you create better health, increased energy, enhanced performance, improved relationships, greater happiness, and more success.

SCHEDULE YOUR 10 MINUTES: Decide what time of day you will practice your heart walk. Morning? Lunch? Evening? Make an appointment with yourself now.

Quick Coherence

Step 1: Heart Focus

Focus your attention on the area of your heart. If this sounds confusing, try this simple exercise. Focus on your right big toe and wiggle it. Now focus on your right elbow. Now, gently focus in the center of your chest, the area of your heart. If you like, you can put your hand over your heart to help. If your mind wanders, just keep shifting your attention back to the area of your heart.

Step 2: Heart Breathing

As you focus on the area of your heart, pretend your breath is flowing in and out through that area. This helps your mind and energy to stay focused in the heart area and your respiration and heart rhythms to synchronize. Breathe slowly and gently, in through your heart (to a count of five or six), and slowly and easily out through your heart (to a count of five or six). Do this until your breathing feels smooth and balanced, not forced. Continue to breathe with ease until you find a natural inner rhythm that feels good to you.

Step 3: Heart Feeling

Continue to breathe through the area of your heart. As you do so, recall a positive feeling, a time when you felt good inside, and try to re-experience it. This could be a feeling of appreciation or care toward a special person or a pet, a place you enjoy or an activity that was fun. Allow yourself to feel this good feeling of appreciation or care. Once you've found a positive feeling or attitude, you can sustain it by continuing your heart focus, heart breathing, and heart feeling. It's that simple.

This technique is also used with a heart-rate coherence software program created by Doc Childre, founder of HeartMath. The program is called the Freeze-Framer (www.freezeframer.com), and it will give you a deeper understanding about the purpose and applications for the technique.

Note: If you are unable to walk for any reason, then simply practice this exercise while riding a stationary bike, practicing yoga, stretching, walking in a pool, or sitting in a chair. Of course, consult your doctor before beginning any exercise routine.

11th-Minute Miracle

Today I open my heart to you, God, and allow all your loving energy to radiate through me. I know your love is always within me, God. I know it is a love that radiates warmth. It is a love that heals, and it is a love that shines contagiously on others. So fill me up with your love, God. I am ready to soak it up and share it with others. I am also ready to cultivate love within myself and multiply it a thousand times through my loving thoughts and loving actions. With love, all miracles are possible.

Energy Foundation Tracker

I ate breakfast.	■
I ate smaller healthy meals and energizing snacks.	■
I drank plenty of water.	■
I slept enough to feel energized and rested.	■
I engaged in some form of physical activity.	■
I listened to energizing music.	■
I connected with people who increase my energy.	■
I practiced my energizer breath when stressed.	■

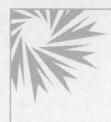

Become a Love Magnet

"Love is the divine force that connects us
to ourselves, each other, and everything
in the universe."

—Jon Gordon

When I am asked, "Jon, how can I find a loving relationship?" or "How can I create a loving marriage?" or "How can I get over not being loved by my parents?" or "How can I get some love from my company in the form of a raise or promotion?" my answer is the same. Become a love magnet. You don't become a love magnet by wearing expensive cologne or perfume, or by getting a new car or hairstyle, or by playing corporate politics. Rather you become a love magnet when you become a source of love—when instead of seeking and craving love, you become the love you already are. Instead of searching for it in other people, you find it within yourself.

Sure, we all want to be loved and have love in our lives, but we'll never find it in others unless we discover it in ourselves first. The world is a mirror, and the love we hope to see out there must be reflected from in here. When you are needy for love, you'll always have to fight and struggle to get it. But when you become a love magnet, you'll attract all the love you could ever want and more. It will flow into your life as a river flows into the ocean. Make your life a haven for love, and like a child who jumps into her/his parents' arms, love will wrap itself around you and never let go. To become a love magnet, it is essential to become a source of love—and this starts by loving yourself, loving others, and cultivating loving emotions. Here are several ways you can become a love magnet.

➤ **Speak lovingly to yourself.** We may be kind to others, but many of us are extremely hard on ourselves. We berate ourselves and undervalue our self-worth. Pay attention to your language, and make sure you are kind to yourself. When you love yourself without arrogance, others will be attracted to you, and more love will flow into your life. Instead of searching for love, try loving yourself and love will find you.

➤ **Treat yourself with love.** Realize you are important. Don't let anyone tell you or cause you to feel otherwise. Then take action by treating yourself with love. Get the massage you don't think you deserve. Take time for yourself every day. Even if it's only 10 minutes. That's what this plan is all about.

➤ **Become love in action.** People always think to get love they have to go after it and find it from others. Actually, the best way to receive love is to share it. When we become a source of love and share it with our families, coworkers, friends, and communities, we become one with all the love that exists and it flows to us with ten times the power and grace. When we give love, we open the dam and love pours into our life. So, today, stop asking how you can get more love from everyone else and start sharing it.

But here's the key—many people give love with attachment and neediness. They think they are giving, but really they are only giving to suck love and energy back. This doesn't make you a magnet. It makes you an energy vampire. Expecting love or being needy for love actually creates resistance and blocks the flow of love in your life. So to be a true love magnet, share love without attachments and expectations. Share your effort and energy without looking over your shoulder to see who is watching. Take action and give of yourself, but don't give to get in return. How do you know the difference? When you give of yourself, you feel energized. When you give to get in return, you feel drained.

➤ **Remember who you are.** When it comes to love, we can't forget to talk about spiritual energy because love and God are one and the same. When you are sharing love, you are expressing the spiritual energy of love that is all around you. When you become a source of love, you become an expression of the greater and greatest source of love. Remember that you are an expression of this source. You came from this source and you are this source. You may not have been loved by your parents, but you have always been part of this source. In remembering this, you realize that the love you have always wanted is already within you waiting to be tapped and expressed.

Now let's put this love into action.

SCHEDULE YOUR 10 MINUTES some time in the morning: Decide when you will do your 10-minute exercise this morning. Schedule your time now. Add it to your calendar or PDA.

Action Steps

➤ Look in the mirror and say, "You are beautiful" or "You are handsome." Then say, "I love you. I really love you." Do this for a few minutes. I know it sounds funny and may feel a little awkward, but it is important to honor yourself and who you are. You don't say, "I love you," from a standpoint of arrogance but rather from a perspective that love's the very essence of who you are. Not the beauty on the outside but the beauty that comes from the very essence of your soul.

➤ Wrap your arms around yourself and give yourself a hug. Again, tell yourself, "I love you."

➤ Rub your fingers through your hair, starting at your forehead and moving over your scalp. Then take your fingers and rub the back of your neck. Doing this reminds you that you deserve attention. You deserve to take care of yourself. You are worthy of your own love and attention. You need it and you deserve it.

➤ Cultivate a feeling of love just as you did during the heart walk yesterday. Think of a time when you felt loved or when you truly loved someone or something.

➤ Share your love with others. Think of various people in your life and send them love through your thoughts. You might think of your mother or a friend and say, "I send you love." You can even do this for a relative or friend who is deceased. As Einstein taught us, from God's perspective there is no such thing as time.

➤ Write down in your journal how you feel.

11th-Minute Miracle

I know that I am loved by you, God. I am an expression of your love, and I was born to share this love with others. I am not my ego or fears. I am love in action, and within me exists all the love in the universe. So today I ask you to help me fill my heart with love. Let me take a bath in your loving energy. Make me a conduit for the love you want to share in the world. Help me to know this love in my own life, and let it spill over to everyone I meet. I am here to improve and grow every day, and I know that love will show me the way. I know that love is a choice and I must make the choice to love. I must make my life a sanctuary for your love. So today I make the commitment to choose love instead of hate. Love instead of fear. Love instead of anger. Love instead of pain. I will cultivate love in my life and become a powerful love magnet.

Energy Foundation Tracker

I ate breakfast.	■
I ate smaller healthy meals and energizing snacks.	■
I drank plenty of water.	■
I slept enough to feel energized and rested.	■
I engaged in some form of physical activity.	■
I listened to energizing music.	■
I connected with people who increase my energy.	■
I practiced my energizer breath when stressed.	■

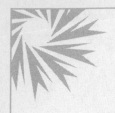

Week 4 Day 27

Cultivate Compassion

"If you want others to be happy, practice compassion. If you want to be happy, practice compassion."

—The Dalai Lama

In the book *Destructive Emotions,* author Daniel Goleman explained that when Buddhist monk Lama Öser was generating a state of compassion during meditation, he showed a remarkable leftward shift in prefrontal cortex activity, indicating a high level of happiness and positive emotion. It appears that when we generate compassion and concern for the well-being of others, we greatly improve our own well-being. Ironically, by generating heartfelt emotions and a genuine concern for others, we may be the ones who benefit most. While we can't personally measure this activity in our own brains without the advanced scientific equipment used on Öser, we can receive the same benefits of cultivating compassion during meditation by performing the same exercises as Öser. When you combine meditation with the act of cultivating love and compassion, you get a powerful exercise that increases your happiness, reduces your stress, creates coherency, and recharges your batteries. And like all the exercises in this plan, compassion doesn't have to take a lot of time. You just have to put yourself in the shoes of others, connect with your heart, and have empathy for those who are suffering. While we are all born with compassion, research shows we can cultivate it by doing exercises like the one you will practice today. Enjoy your 10 minutes of compassion.

SCHEDULE YOUR 10 MINUTES OF COMPASSION today. What time will you take this energy break? Commit to it! Write the time of day or specific time in your journal.

Action Steps
➤ Read the following visualizing exercise.

Close your eyes and visualize someone who is suffering. Perhaps it's a homeless mother or a starving child, a sick relative or a miserable neighbor or coworker. Now visualize a version of yourself as a hateful, selfish, jealous, coldhearted person. Visualize another version of yourself as a neutral observer. Visualize this neutral observer version of yourself standing in the center. Visualize the selfish, hateful version of yourself on your right. And visualize the person who is suffering on your left. As you see this picture, whom do you as the neutral observer gravitate toward? Whom do you want to help? I'm sure it's the homeless mother, starving child, sick relative, or miserable friend.

Then see this person who is suffering. Think about how this suffering might be impacting his or her life. Realize that you don't want this person to suffer. Think about how you want him or her to be free of pain and full of happiness. Think about how you can help this person be free of suffering and help take away the pain.

Now see yourself helping this person. See yourself giving him/her clothes, money, love, and support. See yourself making him/her smile. Then imagine yourself taking away his/her pain. See yourself removing his/her fear, stress, and negative energy. See yourself as a powerful force of positive energy, sharing your energy with someone in need and helping to remove pain and suffering. See yourself as a compassionate, caring, empathetic person making a difference.

➤ Now practice this visualizing exercise. Close your eyes and sit in silence while you cultivate compassion.

➤ After this exercise, write down in your journal how you feel.

11th-Minute Miracle

I surrender my hate and anger to you, God. I surrender the heavy negative energy that clouds my heart and stops me from feeling love and compassion. As I go about my day, God, I ask that you show me the way. Provide me with the strength and patience to practice compassion. Help me recognize the suffering in others. Fill my heart with love. Remind me that I am connected to everyone and everything. Help me to overcome my selfish ego so I may share my energy, compassion, and love with others. Help me become the change I wish to see in the world. Help me turn into the compassionate, loving, and powerful force of energy that I know I am. Help me to be my best self.

Energy Foundation Tracker

I ate breakfast.

I ate smaller healthy meals and energizing snacks.

I drank plenty of water.

I slept enough to feel energized and rested.

I engaged in some form of physical activity.

I listened to energizing music.

I connected with people who increase my energy.

I practiced my energizer breath when stressed.

Week 4 Day 28

Pray for Someone or Something

"If you want happiness for an hour—take a nap. If you want happiness for a day—go fishing. If you want happiness for a month— get married. If you want happiness for a year—inherit a fortune. If you want happiness for a lifetime—help someone else."

—Chinese proverb

One of the ultimate ways to energize yourself and others is by praying. When you pray for someone, you not only increase your health and happiness but, amazingly, you have a positive effect on the people you pray for. By praying for someone, you are asking God, the universe, a higher power, or whatever you call the infinite and timeless source of energy from which everything emanates, to heal this person of their suffering or illness. When you pray for someone, you use the power of your thoughts and words and intention to help another person—which is truly a selfless and compassionate act. And the most amazing thing about prayer is that it really does work.

Prayer is so powerful that 79 of the nation's 125 medical schools now offer courses on prayer and spirituality. According to Larry Dossey, M.D., an expert on spirituality and medicine, researchers have conducted approximately two hundred scientific studies on prayer and health. About two-thirds of these studies have shown positive results in patients with chest pain, heart attack, and AIDS. Amazingly, people who are prayed for are more likely to recover than those who are not prayed for.

Prayer is definitely good medicine for others and it is definitely good for you, too. Research suggests that those with a strong spiritual faith live longer and happier lives, are more likely to overcome adversity, and recover faster and stronger from heart and hip surgeries. Prayer is the ultimate energizer. So what can you do? You can sit in silence to recharge your batteries. While sitting in silence, you can pray for someone and engage in the ultimate act of compassion. Through your prayer exercise, you can develop spiritual muscle for a long and happy life.

TODAY SCHEDULE YOUR 10 MINUTES OF PRAYER and pray for someone who needs your help. Schedule your 10 minutes now.

Action Steps

➤ Find a comfortable and quiet place.

➤ Identify which person or people you are going to pray for. Write their names in your journal if you wish.

➤ Now get comfortable and sit in silence for a few minutes. Focus on the sensations of your body to help you focus and relax. Listen to your breath. Feel your heartbeat. Feel the air touch your skin.

➤ Then spend the rest of your time praying for those whom you want to help with your prayers. If they are sick, pray that they be healed. Pray for their highest good and their best outcome. If they are in emotional pain, pray that they will be free of suffering. Pray that they will know joy and happiness in their life instead of fear and despair. Pray that they will be happy, healthy, successful, and confident. Pray that a family member will get through a difficult time. Pray that a family member will find a healthy and happy relationship.

➤   Write in your journal how you feel after you have finished praying.

11th-Minute Miracle

I trust in you, God. I know you will always be with me. You will walk within my step. You will breathe within my breath. You will shine within my light. You will love within my embrace. I know you are the whisper that moves me in the right direction. You are the voice in my dreams that says, "You can do it." You are the arm that lifts me up when I fall. You are the nudge that tells me to "get going." You are the goose bumps that alert me to the truth. You are the love in my heart. And you are the light that shines inside me. So thank you for expressing your love through me. Thank you for teaching me to be a better person. Thank you for all the experiences I have had and will have. Thank you for providing me with a roof over my head and food to eat. Thank you for the hands to write, legs to walk, and mouth to talk. Thank you for the opportunity to improve my life and thank you for the love, joy, and happiness that is all around me. Thank you for the 11th-Minute Miracle. I look forward to seeing and experiencing all the miracles in my life.

Energy Foundation Tracker

I ate breakfast.	▪
I ate smaller healthy meals and energizing snacks.	▪
I drank plenty of water.	▪
I slept enough to feel energized and rested.	▪

I engaged in some form of physical activity.   ▪

I listened to energizing music.   ▪

I connected with people who increase my energy.   ▪

I practiced my energizer breath when stressed.   ▪

Week 4

Evaluation—
Where Are You Now?

You've completed the fourth week of the plan. Only two days left to go. Do you feel more alive, more focused, more positive? Complete the following scales, and let me know how you are doing. I would love to hear from you. E-mail me at jon@jongordon.com. Also visit me at www.jongordon.com to receive an energy boost for the final week of the plan.

Negative Energy–Positive Energy Scale

1	2	3	4	5	6	7	8	9	10

Negative   Positive

Sad-Happy Scale

1	2	3	4	5	6	7	8	9	10

Sad   Happy

Stressed Scale

1	2	3	4	5	6	7	8	9	10

Stressed   Relaxed

Focused Scale

1	2	3	4	5	6	7	8	9	1 0

Scattered   Focused

Fear-Trust Scale

1	2	3	4	5	6	7	8	9	1 0

Fear   Trust

Overall Energy Scale

1	2	3	4	5	6	7	8	9	1 0

Low   High

Chapter 9

The 10-Minute-a-Day Plan—Days 29 and 30

Give Someone Else 10 Minutes of Energy

One of the best ways to find happiness and meaning in your own life is to make a difference in someone else's. And one of the best ways to increase your energy is by sharing your positive energy with someone else. Energy does not decrease when it's shared, but rather it multiplies with each act of love and kindness. Thus, during the last two days of the plan you will give someone else 10 minutes of your energy. You will engage in acts of compassion, kindness, and gratitude, and in doing so you will not only benefit others but yourself as well. According to Howard Cutler, author of *The Art of Happiness,* "In a study by James House of the University of Michigan Research Center, researchers discovered that engaging in regular volunteer activities and interacting with others in a compassionate way dramatically increased life expectancy and probably overall vitality as well." Compassionate actions are not only good for the world, but they are also good for you.

Research also shows that kindness is an antidepressant. Those who are the recipient of an act of kindness produce more serotonin.

Those who engage in the act of kindness also produce more serotonin, and even those who watch the act of kindness produce more serotonin. So by sharing kindness, you in essence create your own antidepressant factory. And best of all, these antidepressants are free.

By giving someone else 10 minutes of energy you will both give and receive the gift of positive energy. Positive energy is contagious, so share it and let it grow.

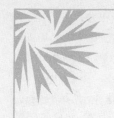

Day 29

Give the Gift
of Kindness

In the natural order of things, systems, organizations, and groups that communicate with one another, help one another, and share with one another are healthier and more likely to survive than those that don't. Just imagine a group of ants that didn't work together, or a society where no one cooperated with one another, or even a group of cells in your body that didn't communicate with the rest of the body. (This leads to cancer).

It is no surprise then that a key part of our survival and happiness is kindness and engaging and receiving in acts of kindness. The plain truth is that we need one another. No man or woman is an island of energy, stranded by themselves in the middle of a huge ocean. We are all part of the collective energy that lights the stars, fires up the sun, and makes the world go round. We are all little pieces of energy that contribute to the whole sea of life. Just as it is essential for each one of our cells to communicate and share information and resources with one another to maintain our health, it is essential for us to help and communicate with one another to maintain not only the health of our outer world but our inner world as well. At our core we are creatures who are born to be kind, and when we practice kindness, we increase our health and happiness.

At the University of California at Riverside, psychologist Sonja Lyubomirsky researched different techniques and strategies that increase our happiness. Not surprisingly one of the successful happiness boosters is performing acts of kindness—such as volunteering for a charity, opening the door for someone, feeding the homeless, or taking elderly neighbors grocery shopping. Lyubomirsky has found that by engaging in five acts of kindness in a single day, participants in her studies experience a measurable boost in happiness. By helping others, we may be the ones who benefit most.

And the great thing about acts of kindness is that they don't have to take up your entire day. They can be short, meaningful, heartfelt acts of kindness that take a minute or two. Sure, if you can spend an entire day at a homeless shelter, that would be wonderful. But don't let a lack of time make you think you can't make a difference in the world or within yourself. By engaging in just five acts of kindness that take up a total of 10 minutes, you can shine your light on your community and within yourself. So today, as you near the end of this thirty-day plan, the goal is to boost your energy and happiness by boosting the energy and happiness of someone else. Practice the following action steps and get out there and share some kindness.

Action Steps

➤ Think about your life and your daily schedule and identify simple ways you can engage in acts of kindness. Think of random acts that may come up and acts that can be planned. For ideas visit www.giftofkindness.com. Write a few of these ideas in your journal.

➤ Commit to engaging in two of these acts today. In other words, two of your five acts of kindness will be planned. This means that three of your kindness acts will be random today. These acts may be the ones you listed above, or they likely will be random acts that present themselves to you during the course of your day—acts you haven't even thought of.

➤ So as you go about your day today, look for opportunities to engage in random acts of kindness. By focusing on sharing kindness and placing your attention on kindness, you will attract more situations and opportunities to be kind. When an act takes place, it will feel like catching a foul ball at a Major League baseball game. Random, but special and wonderful.

➤ Take action, and if more than five acts of kindness should present themselves to you today, then do them and keep the positive energy flowing. Positive energy never decreases by being shared. Rather, with each gift, it grows exponentially greater than the power of a thousand stars.

➤ At the end of the day, write in your journal how it felt to engage in these acts of kindness.

11th-Minute Miracle

I've been asking for you to send me a miracle, God, and you have been sending them. So I just want to thank you. I love the amazing miracles you keep presenting in my life, and I'm ready for whatever you think I need. I am ready for a miracle, and I realize that they happen in your time, not my time. So I'll be patient. Most important, God, I realize that my life is a miracle. I realize that I am a miracle. While I have known struggles, fear, doubt, and pain, I also know that there is a miracle in all of it. I know that the fact that I am here reading these words, breathing this air, and living this life is truly a miracle. Amen.

Energy Foundation Tracker

I ate breakfast.	■
I ate smaller healthy meals and energizing snacks.	■

I drank plenty of water.

I slept enough to feel energized and rested.

I engaged in some form of physical activity.

I listened to energizing music.

I connected with people who increase my energy.

I practiced my energizer breath when stressed.

Day 30

Make a Gratitude Visit

"Like a wilting flower that craves sunlight
and water, humans need positive energy
to grow, flourish, and stand tall above
the weeds."

—Jon Gordon

Martin Seligman, a professor of psychology at the University of Pennsylvania, author of *Authentic Happiness,* and the father of positive psychology, says the most powerful way to supercharge and boost your happiness is to make a "gratitude visit." A gratitude visit is when you write a letter thanking someone who has made a difference in your life, and then you visit this person and read the letter in person. According to Seligman, the amazing thing about this strategy is that "people who do this just once are measurably happier and less depressed a month later."

Whether it's because we are connecting with someone who has helped give our life meaning, or whether the act of writing the letter and sharing it with someone special gives meaning to our life, happiness experts agree that this strategy increases happiness, boosts joy, and causes us to pause and remember what is important in life. Instead of thinking about where we want to go next in our life, a gratitude visit allows us to remember where we have been and recognize the people who helped us along the way. The gratitude visit provides us with a positive remembrance of our past, and this fuels our present life with positive energy and positive meaning. Life is all about moments and memories, and when we take the time to recall great memories, moments, and people, we receive an incredible energy boost. Remember that two thoughts cannot occupy your mind at the same time. So if you are being grateful, you won't be feeling sorry for yourself. Instead of thinking of things that drain your energy, you'll be thinking of people who energize you. Not to mention the incredible positive energy boost received by the person on the receiving end of the gratitude visit.

Just imagine if everyone made gratitude visits a part of their life. We would have rays of positive energy criss-crossing our communities, businesses, cities, and countries. We would have mothers and daughters connecting. Old bosses and mentors would know they made the difference. Students would reconnect with their teachers. And I would make a visit to Tony Cozza, Ivan Goldfarb, and Richard Moran, three people who guided me to Cornell University and changed the course of my life. Through gratitude visits we would create a circular flow of positive energy, giving one day and receiving the next. We would have people knowing that they make a difference in someone's life.

But remember, giving happiness and positive energy is not a one-time event. Seligman says that the effects of a gratitude visit wear off after a few months. Probably a good thing, since if we want to keep receiving the benefits of a gratitude visit, we will make more visits. This will benefit not only us but the world. The positive energy we share affects everyone in our wake, and everyone who comes into contact with those in our wake, until the entire ocean of energy is impacted by you. The love you share today fertilizes the hearts and souls of others, producing bountiful harvests for generations to come. My hope is that after you experience the energy boost of a 10-minute gratitude visit, you will make it a monthly event and continue to receive the benefits of sharing positive energy. But it starts with you and it starts right now.

SCHEDULE YOUR 10-MINUTE GRATITUDE VISIT. At this time you might be saying, "Hey, Jon, I want to make a gratitude visit to a relative in New York and I live in California. This isn't possible right now." Since you may not be able to make a gratitude visit to the person you would most like to visit, for this exercise and this plan the goal is to make a gratitude visit with someone in close proximity to you.

Action Steps

➤ Call up the person you want to thank and schedule a time to get together. Seligman says don't tell them why you want to get together. He believes that surprise makes the gratitude visit even more effective. Write a letter thanking this person for something they have done that made a difference in your life. Then visit this person and take up to 10 minutes to read the letter to them.

➤ If it is impossible to make a gratitude visit, then still write a gratitude letter and make a gratitude call. Read the letter to them over the phone. Although it is not as powerful as being in the same room with the person you are thanking, it is still very powerful and effective.

➤ After your gratitude visit or call, write down in your journal how you feel.

➤ The next time you take a trip to be with someone who lives far away but whom you want to thank, remember to write a gratitude letter, bring it with you, and read it to them when you get together.

➤ Practice gratitude visits and gratitude calls once a month beyond this plan. In the next chapter, we'll talk about this and other ways to keep the energy flowing for the rest of your life.

11th-Minute Miracle

God, as I finish this plan, I pray for the dedication to continue practicing the exercises that have made a difference in my life. I pray for the focus to continue investing 10 minutes a day in myself. I pray that I will continue to make further improvements, minute to minute, day to day, week to week, and year to year. And when I experience challenges, I pray for the ability to use my new skills to flow through life rather than struggle. Use me, God, to help make this world a better place. Begin with me so that I will become the change you want to see. Guide me, God, and have me be what you want me to be and do what you want me to do. Inspire me, God, so I will be filled with your contagious energy. Most of all, thank you, God, for the life I have been given. I will make the most of it.

Energy Foundation Tracker

I ate breakfast.	■
I ate smaller healthy meals and energizing snacks.	■
I drank plenty of water.	■
I slept enough to feel energized and rested.	■
I engaged in some form of physical activity.	■
I listened to energizing music.	■
I connected with people who increase my energy.	■
I practiced my energizer breath when stressed.	■

Measuring Muscle
at Day 30—
Where Are You Now?

You've completed the plan. So how was it? Do you feel more alive, more focused, more positive? Complete the following scales, and let me know how you are doing. I would love to hear from you. E-mail me at jon@jongordon.com

Negative Energy–Positive Energy Scale

| 1 | 2 | 3 | 4 | 5 | 6 | 7 | 8 | 9 | 10 |

Negative   Positive

Sad-Happy Scale

| 1 | 2 | 3 | 4 | 5 | 6 | 7 | 8 | 9 | 10 |

Sad   Happy

Stressed Scale

| 1 | 2 | 3 | 4 | 5 | 6 | 7 | 8 | 9 | 10 |

Stressed   Relaxed

Focused Scale

1	2	3	4	5	6	7	8	9	1 0

Scattered   Focused

Fear-Trust Scale

1	2	3	4	5	6	7	8	9	1 0

Fear   Trust

Overall Energy Scale

1	2	3	4	5	6	7	8	9	1 0

Low   High

Also ask yourself the following questions:

➤ How do you feel?

➤ Do you feel more in control of your emotions? How?

➤ Are you more calm? How?

➤ Has your stress dissipated?

➤ Are you happier?

➤ Do you have more energy?

➤ Do you feel more confident?

➤ Are you more positive?

➤ Are you handling stress better?

➤ Are you more aware of your thoughts?

➤ Are you stronger?

➤ Are you more focused?

➤ Are you more productive?

➤ Do you feel more grateful?

➤ Are you replacing fear with trust?

➤ Are you making better choices for your health, happiness, and energy?

10 Minutes a Day for the Rest of Your Life

How to Keep the Positive Energy Flowing After the 30 Days Are Over

You've completed the plan and you may be wondering, "What should I do now?" Well, as I said earlier in the book, the 10-Minute Energy Solution is not a quick fix approach (in spite of the name!), and this is not meant to be just a thirty-day plan. My goal is that the powerful results you have experienced this past month will inspire you to use these 10-minute exercises for the rest of your life. My hope is that you will continue improving your life so you can feel even better than you do now. After all, if you have noticed improvements in yourself after just thirty days, think about the happiness, abundance, and energy you can create by practicing 10 minutes a day for the rest of your life.

In my seminars I often tell the participants that I'm not here to just motivate them. Motivation doesn't last. People get pumped up, and then, within a few days, the energy is gone. They are left with the question, "Now what?" I tell folks what I am here to do is to inspire them to make changes that will benefit them for the rest of their life.

I don't want to be the shot of adrenaline in anyone's arm. Otherwise people will always need me beside them to give them a shot of energy. Instead, I want to give you the recipe to make your own energy any time you need it. Practicing exercises 10 minutes a day is this recipe.

The reality is that we are either growing or dying every day. It's a part of evolution and our human existence. Use a muscle and it grows. Let it sit in a cast for a month and it will atrophy. The same goes for our mental, emotional, and spiritual muscle. If we don't continue to build it, our minds will become lazy, emotional fat will accumulate, and we will fall back into old habits. Considering the world we live in, this can be very dangerous, since mental, emotional, and spiritual muscle is what we need today to flow and thrive through life's challenges. Just as crossword puzzles and active learning keep your mind sharp, practicing 10 minutes a day will help you continue to build trust, happiness, and positive energy while reducing stress. You have already started building the muscle you need to live a happier, more energetic, positive, calm, and peaceful life. You have the momentum. Now you just have to continue building and growing 10 minutes at a time. To help you incorporate 10 minutes a day into the rest of your life, I want to offer a few suggestions and tools to help you create success.

1. **Restart the plan.** If you are someone who likes and needs structure and a plan to follow, simply restart the plan and begin tomorrow with day 1. When you finish another thirty days, start over again.

2. **Plan a 10-minute exercise for each day.** Each day, choose your favorite exercise or the exercise you need most and schedule it. Write down the action steps. Write your own eleventh-minute miracle or use one from this plan. Complete your energy foundation tracker.

Make a copy of the following to help you plan each day. Or simply use computer paper or download your 10-Minute-a-Day Planner from my website at www.jongordon.com/10 minutesplanner.

10-Minute Exercise _____

Schedule it: _____

Action Steps (Write down specific action steps, or go back through the book and write down the page number that includes the action steps for this exercise.)

11th-Minute Miracle (Write your own here if you like.)

_____

_____

_____

_____

_____

Energy Foundation Tracker

I ate breakfast.   ■

I ate smaller healthy meals and energizing snacks.   ■

I drank plenty of water.	■
I slept enough to feel energized and rested.	■
I engaged in some form of physical activity.	■
I listened to energizing music.	■
I connected with people who increase my energy.	■
I practiced my energizer breath when stressed.	■

3. **Practice energy building.** Pick one 10-minute-a-day exercise and just do that exercise every day until it becomes a habit. Then, when it truly feels like a part of your life, add another 10-minute exercise to your schedule. When the second 10-minute exercise becomes a habit, add a third exercise. For example, you may start off with a positive energy exercise every morning. Then, when it becomes a habit, add a 10-minute Thank-You Walk to your schedule and take this walk every day after lunch. Once this becomes a habit, you may decide to practice 10 Minutes of Silent Energy every day when you come home from work. Eventually, you will have incorporated three or more 10-minute exercises into your life, which will help you create amazing results and a powerful life.

   Pick the three exercises you want to incorporate into your life. Choose them in the order in which you will practice them, and list them in your journal.

Use the Ritual Planner to schedule your 10-minute exercises. Here's an example, using the scenario I mentioned above.

10-Minute Exercise	Action	Time(s)	Days
1. 10 Minutes of Positive Energy	Positive Energy Walk	7:30 a.m. to 7:40 a.m.	Monday–Sunday
2. 10 Minutes of Happiness	Thank-You Walk	Lunchtime	Monday–Friday
3. 10 Minutes of Silent Energy	Meditate	6 p.m. after work	Monday–Friday

Use the planner below, or visit www.jongordon.com/ritualplanner and download as many copies as you like.

10-Minute Exercise	Action	Time(s)	Days
1.			
2.			
3.			

4. **Create your own 10-minute exercises.** After practicing the exercises I created for you, I bet you will think of some great 10-minute exercises of your own. Definitely give them a try and see how they work for you. I would also love to hear about your

ideas and results. E-mail me at jon@jongordon.com. Of course, if I share these exercises with others, I will credit you.

5. **Continue practicing the 11th-Minute Miracle.** When I had a thousand people try this plan before I decided to write this book, many selected the 11th-minute miracle as their favorite part of the plan. In this spirit I encourage you to write your own 11th-minute miracles. Write them, read them, and then say them aloud. Share them with others. Share them with me. I would love to read them. E-mail me at jon@jongordon.com. Or if you want me to write more of them, let me know. I am thinking about writing a daily devotional titled *The 11th-Minute Miracle*. What do you think?

Flow with Purpose and Strength

In addition to continuing the 10-Minute-a-Day Plan, there is one final and essential tip I must share with you to help you keep the positive energy flowing throughout the rest of your life. I chose to save it until now because it's the last thing I want you to remember, and it may be the most important. The most powerful way to live a more energetic, happy, rewarding, and meaningful life is to *identify your strengths and use them to serve a cause greater than yourself*. While this sounds simple, I can attest that from all the people I have coached, and through my own life experiences, it is something many of us fail to do.

As I shared at the start of this book, I know this from firsthand experience. For several years I floundered, unhappy and miserable with my life, until my wife told me she was going to leave me if I didn't change. That one moment caused me to ask myself, "What am I good at, what are my strengths, and what was I born to do? Why was I put here on earth?" From that moment on, I started applying my strengths in my life, and my mission was to energize millions of people one person at a time. I found my cause, and I have never enjoyed life more or felt more energized than I do now. Martin Seligman calls this "living the meaningful life," and he believes it is essential to lasting happiness. I believe it is also essential for lasting energy, because purpose is the ultimate fuel for our work and life. While projects, money, prestige, and goals often provide you with incentives in the short term, eventually projects are finished, money is made or lost, prestige comes and goes, and goals are achieved or forgotten. The question is "What then?" People often ask me, "Where does one find the passion, excitement, and energy to stay motivated and energized for the long term?" I tell them that only purpose can do this. Purpose is like a candle that doesn't stop burning. It sustains you during the tough times, and it is with you when the applause stops.

When we have a purpose, we engage with life and with people. We look forward to getting out of bed in the morning. We enjoy doing what we do each day. We live and work with enthusiasm. We have a reason to take on and overcome daily obstacles. We get into the flow of life. When we have a purpose, we apply our energy and strengths toward a cause greater than our own.

In the following and final exercise of this plan, you will identify your strengths and take action steps to develop and live your purpose. Note, however, that if you are someone who says, "I have no idea what my purpose is and I don't know what my strengths are," I encourage you to simply start asking yourself, "What are my strengths?" and "What is my purpose?" Don't force answers. Don't expect results. Just start putting your attention on discovering your strengths and asking your purpose to find you. People are often surprised that I tell them to let their purpose find them, but I have found when we ask and are silent, waiting without expectations, the answers often appear. To discover your strengths, you may also want to ask your close friends and coworkers to identify your strengths. This may point you in an amazing new direction.

Another way to find your purpose is to not think of your purpose as some perfect magical, fairy-tale, unattainable purpose but to realize that we can find meaning and purpose in everyday life. No matter what job we have or what role we play in life, everything can become mundane and ordinary if we let it. For example, a career as an actor, which seems so exciting to the outside world, can become very monotonous to an actor who has lost his passion and purpose. The same goes for a speaker who is just going through the motions or a call center sales representative who gets tired of talking on the phone. The key is that we have to find the purpose in what we do everyday. We must find the extraordinary in the ordinary. The passion in the mundane.

When the newness of any new job wears off, you must ask yourself, *What is my purpose and what can I do to make a difference?* Perhaps you are a cashier and your purpose is to make each person smile as he or she leaves the store. Or maybe you're a doctor and your purpose is to keep every patient healthy. When you find the purpose in the everyday, you will be engaged in life, and thus your ultimate purpose and passion will find you. As you complete the following action steps, you will see that purpose can be found everywhere—from big dreams to small acts of kindness. Once you find it, use it as an ever-flowing source of fuel for your life.

So use this final exercise to help you identify your strengths and live your purpose. Practice your 10-Minute-a-Day Exercises, use your strengths, live a meaningful life, and watch your happiness and energy soar.

Apply Your Strengths and Fuel Up with Purpose

1. First identify your strengths. What are your skills? What are you good at?

- _____
- _____
- _____
- _____
- _____

2. Identify several ways you can start using your strengths at work.

- _____
- _____
- _____

3. If it is not possible to use your strengths at work at this time, then identify what hobby or side business would allow you to use your strengths.

- _____
- _____
- _____

4. Take action.

5. Now, fuel up with purpose. Let's try to discover it first.

Values

Adventure	Balance *(work & home)*	Communication	Community
Commitment	Compassion	Creativity	Dignity
Empathy	Energy	Enthusiasm	Ethics

Excellence	Fairness	Faith	Family
Forgiveness	Friendship	Generosity	Genuineness
Harmony	Health	Honesty	Humor/Fun
Initiative	Integrity	Joy	Knowledge
Leadership	Learning	Loyalty	Making a difference
Other people	Peace	Positive Energy	Responsibility
Success	Teamwork	Trust	Wisdom

➤ To find purpose, first identify the top five values and characteristics that matter most to you. To find purpose in something, you have to value it. Please choose from the list above or come up with your own.

1._____   4. _____

2._____   5._____

3._____

➤ If you passed away today and someone gave a eulogy at your funeral, what would you want them to say about you?

_____

_____

➤ Pretend you are a newspaper reporter, and write a few sentences about yourself. The article would be sent to your friends, family, and associates. What nice things would the article say about you?

_____

_____

_____

_____

_____

➤ If you found out that tomorrow was the last day of your life, what life lessons would you want to share with your children or grandchildren?

1._____

2._____

3._____

4._____

➤ Now do a reality check. Are you living your values? Are you incorporating your strengths into your life? Are you applying the lessons that you would want to share with your children or grandchildren? Are you the person the reporter described? If any of the answers are "no," then write down what's missing. For example, one of your values might be family. However, answering these questions makes you realize that you don't spend any time with your family. Thus, spending time with family would be missing from your life.

_____

_____

➤ Through these exercises you will hopefully find the missing purposes in your life. While you may be living some of your purposes, what's often missing is the purpose and fuel you need most. For example, one of the lessons you might want to share with your future generations is to make a difference in other people's lives. Yet you find yourself often being distant and unfriendly with friends and strangers. Thus, one of your missing purposes might be to make one person's day every day. Write your purposes here.

1._____

2._____

3._____

4._____

➤ Once you discover your purposes, the key is to incorporate them into your life. Life and work offer a tremendous amount of opportunity to live your purposes. We just have to find the deeper meaning in everyday things. When you connect your everyday life with your values, beliefs, and convictions, you fuel up with purpose.

For example, even if you don't love your job, try to find purpose in it. Perhaps it's something as simple as creating positive interactions. Or find your purpose after work. My friend Amy felt her purpose was to make people laugh. As a pharmaceuticals rep and comedian, she makes doctors laugh by day and audiences laugh by night. So, connect your purpose to your everyday personal and professional life.

➤ Write down one statement of purpose for your professional life. For example, you might write, "My purpose is to develop my employees into successful leaders. I spend the time and effort to train them. I am patient when they make mistakes. I set high expectations so they strive for the very best."

_____

_____

_____

_____

➤ Now write down several rituals that will help you live this purpose. For example, one ritual for the statement of purpose above
  might be, "Personal Development Seminar." The action would
  be "listening to a speaker once a month on Mondays."

	Ritual	Action	Time(s)	Days
1.				
2.				
3.				

➤ Write down one statement of purpose for your personal life. For
  example, you might write, "My purpose is to raise my children
  into happy, strong, compassionate, and successful adults."

_____

_____

_____

_____

➤ Now write down several rituals that will help you live this purpose. For example, one ritual for the statement of purpose above might be, "Read each night to my children." The action would be to "read books that teach morals each night at eight, Monday through Friday."

	Ritual	Action	Time(s)	Days
1.				
2.				
3.				

Power Statement *(Say this daily)*:

Each day I choose to live a life filled with meaning and purpose. This provides me with sustained energy for the short term and long term.

Share the
Energy

As you have come to realize in reading this book, positive energy is contagious—and my mission is not only to help you find more energy for your life and career but also to help you share your positive energy with others. When we become "positively contagious," we create an energy flow that changes our families, our communities, our world, and ourselves. Some people call it idealistic to think that one person can have such an impact. I call it obvious, when you understand the laws of energy. The collective energy of our world is created by the individual expression and energy of each person who lives on this planet.

To change our communities, our society, our country, and our planet, we must first change ourselves. We must become, as Gandhi said, "the change we wish to see in the world." Once we become this change, then we can help others become this change by first being a living and walking example of this change. We teach best by example. As St. Francis said, "It's no use walking anywhere to preach unless your walking is your preaching." By walking our walk, we can share this positive energy, one person at a time. As we do this in our towns and communities, positive energy will spread faster than any gossip or flu bug. Every moment of every day we have a choice—to share positive energy or negative energy. We can share fear or trust, hate or love, gossip or meaningful stories. Change happens one moment, one action, and one interaction at a time. To help foster this change, I want to introduce you to several of my initiatives and resources that will help you cultivate positive energy within yourself and allow you to share it with others.

PEP (Positive Energy Program)

PEP is my nonprofit 501C3 initiative that helps parents and teachers develop healthy, positive kids. PEP is a whole solution that works with all the people involved in raising and teaching whole children. PEP provides physical, mental, and emotional development strategies, actions plans, lesson plans, and programs for parents, teachers, and school systems. Our programs develop strong bodies, strong minds, and emotional power. PEP also helps schools cultivate more positive energy. Teachers become more energized and focused, students become more positive and healthy, and parents become more involved and focused.

Visit www.positiveenergyprogram.com for:

➤ A free 7-Step Plan to raise healthy, positive kids
➤ Lesson plans for teachers
➤ Resources for parents

Energy Mastery Program

This is my twelve-month course for people who want to increase their mental, physical, emotional, and spiritual energy. This year of energy course includes:

➤ Weekly teleclasses (lectures over the phone), strategies, take-home exercises, and action steps to help transform your energy, health, happiness, and life

➤ Online resources, lessons, and strategies based on the latest research in self-improvement

➤ Access to my coaching center, filled with audio tips, teleconferences, CDs, and course materials

➤ Live Q&A sessions after each teleclass where you can receive answers to your most pressing issues and questions

➤ Guest lectures with the greatest minds in the field of health, happiness, wellness, self-improvement, and success

➤ Group support via our message boards

➤ Updates from me regarding my latest research and insights

➤ 2-Day Energy Retreat

Visit www.energymasterprogram.com for more information about the Energy Mastery Program.

Energy Coach University

Because I have had so many requests from people who want to learn how to become an energy coach, I have created Energy Coach University. If you are a psychotherapist, counselor, life coach, physical trainer, or chiropractor who wants to learn how to become an energy coach, Energy Coach University offers a fifteen-month intensive training program.

Visit www.energycoachuniversity.com for more information.

Chief Energy Officer Training Programs

Energy is the currency of personal and company success. It is the foundation of emotional intelligence, contagious leadership, inspired customer service, and team effectiveness. Chief energy officers utilize energy to develop powerful customer relationships, grow profits, boost company morale, and enhance productivity. They overcome adversity and challenges to create success, and they share positive contagious energy with their customers, coworkers, and employees. And the great thing is that anyone can become chief energy officer. You don't have to be the CEO to be the chief energy officer. Since energy is essential to a happy and successful life, I created the chief energy officer to help all the people who are drained in the corporate world—and there are a lot of them. I've worked with hundreds of companies and thousands of employees, and this program makes a difference.

Visit www.chiefenergyofficer.com for more information.

3-Day Energy Retreat

Come to my energy center, at the oceanfront Ponte Vedra Inn and Club, and we'll spend three days learning and creating strategies, routines, and a plan to enhance your health, happiness, energy, and success. Whether you want to take your life or career, or both, to the next level . . . we'll do it together. For three days we will work together to identify where you are, determine where you want to go, and create and implement a plan that will help you get there. Along the way I will teach you, guide you, inspire you, and help you stay focused, positive, and on track. Together we'll identify those of your thoughts and beliefs that are helping you build your life and those causing you to tear your life down; discover powerful techniques and strategies to enhance every aspect of your life and career; build physical health and vibrancy; reduce stress; increase your happiness and positive energy; unleash your joy and purpose; let go of what is holding you back; and create meaningful interactions with other seminar participants.

Visit www.jongordon.com for more information, or call 904-285-6842 for more information.

Grow the Energy

10-Minute-a-Day Resources

If this book has infected you with a positive energy bug, then I want to help you keep the momentum going with additional resources that will further support, encourage, and inspire you. I have put together a series of resources that will help you on your path to mental, emotional, and spiritual growth. Understand that you don't have to read everything at once. Growth is a process. Just take your time and soak up everything you can. Like the sun, let these books, Web sites, magazines, and other resources be a source of fuel that energizes your life. Books are energy and the words, thoughts, and ideas we take into our consciousness determine the future of our lives.

Books

*Energy Addict: 101 Physical, Mental, and Spiritual Ways to
   Energize Your Life* by Jon Gordon
Destructive Emotions by Daniel Goleman
An Open Heart by the Dalai Lama
The HeartMath Solution by Doc Childre and Howard Martin

Heart of the Soul by Gary Zukov
Seat of the Soul by Gary Zukov
Everyday Grace by Marianne Williamson
The Power of Intention by Wayne Dyer
The Field by Lynne McTaggart
The Art of Happiness by Howard Cutler and the Dalai Lama
What Happy People Know by Dan Baker
The Greatest Salesman by Og Mandino
Illusions by Richard Bach
Quantum Healing by Deepak Chopra
The Power of Now by Eckhart Tolle

Websites

www.jongordon.com
www.positivepsychology.org
www.reflectivehappiness.com
www.drweil.com
www.chopra.com
www.spiritualcinemacircle.com
www.giftofkindness.com
www.endfatigue.com

Magazines

O, The Oprah Magazine
Prevention
Shift from Noetic Sciences
Body and Soul
Organic Style
Spirituality and Health
Health
Men's Health

INDEX

About the Author

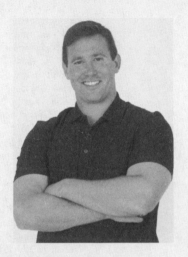

Jon Gordon is the author of *Energy Addict* and is a popular speaker, workshop leader, and energy coach. He has appeared on NBC's *Today* show and has also been featured in *Men's Health, Self, Woman's Day, Redbook,* and hundreds of other print, television, and online media. He coaches thousands of individuals and organizations each year, including the PGA Tour, the Jacksonville Jaguars, Wachovia Bank, Chubb Insurance, Cingular Wireless, GE, State Farm Insurance, the United Way, and the Super Bowl Host Committee. He lives in northeast Florida with his wife and two children. Visit him and sign up for your free weekly energy tip at www.jongordon.com.

Visit Jon's Website at

www.jongordon.com

- ➤ Receive Jon's free weekly energy tip.
- ➤ Download the *10-Minute Energy Solution* planning pages.
- ➤ Ask Jon questions about the plan.
- ➤ Listen to Jon's weekly messages to guide you through the plan.
- ➤ Find out when Jon will be in your city or town.
- ➤ Connect with others who are using the plan.
- ➤ Share the positive energy.

I want to hear your 10-Minute
Energy Solution Success Stories!

Has the plan helped you? What did
you like best about it? What was
your biggest transformation?
Did you have an *aha* moment during
the plan? Do you have any
suggestions?

I would love to hear from you!

E-mail me at jon@jongordon.com.

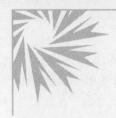

Acknowledgments

I would like to thank the following people for helping make this book possible. Because of them I have been able to live my mission of energizing as many people as possible, one person at a time.

My wife and children, for making me feel like the luckiest man on earth.

My parents, for making me feel like a success every day of my life.

Daniel Decker, my chief energy officer. I call him MacGyver for a reason. He always finds a way to make it happen, and there is nothing he can't do. He joined me at a time when all I had was a vision, and he helped me turn this vision into reality.

Arielle Ford and Brian Hilliard, for being my adviser and friend. Without them this book would not have happened. I will be forever grateful to them.

Michelle Howry, my incredible editor, who is somehow always on the same wavelength with me. Her amazing editing and magical touch helped me create a book that I believe will make a difference in many people's lives. I am so grateful for her support, guidance, and ideas that improved every facet of this book.

John Duff, for seeing my vision and helping me make this book possible.

Kerry Byrnes, for helping me share my energy and tips with the NBC *Today* show viewers.

Mark and Janice Rathjen, for our fateful reunion that would change my life forever.

Vince Bagni, for being a good friend and a terrific energy ambassador.

Shawn O'Shell, for his incredible graphics and design.

Emilie Pennington and Francis Ablola, for helping me spread the positive energy.

Susan Turnbull, for giving her time and energy to help those who need more energy, hope, and purpose in their life.

All my newsletter subscribers, for sharing the positive energy and finding the strength to overcome life's challenges and obstacles. I admire you.